Advance Praise for *Miriam's Secret:*

"An inspirational healing book, reaching out to the deep feminine well of wisdom at the heart of a shared tradition. Eliana Gilad is an extraordinary musician, reconnecting Miriam's Exodus music and leadership with Hathor's ecstatic goddess cult in ancient Egypt."
—**Alison Roberts,** author of *Hathor Rising*

"What a wonderful, well researched, musical invitation to step into the story of the Promised Land! I highly recommend it."
—**Christine Stevens,** author of *Music as Medicine*

"*Miriam's Secret* is a brilliant book providing spiritual signposts from ancient Israel that point toward people leading a meaningful life where they can truly pursue their passions and enjoy the journey. I highly recommend it for anyone on a spiritual search to discover his or her inner wisdom. Eliana Gilad establishes an authoritative study of ancient Israel and feminine wisdom culture, and develops a dialogue that inspires the soul towards true transformation."
—**Justin St. Vincent,** author of *Spiritual Significance of Music*

I wish you both the deepening of your wisdom & a beautiful connection to the Source of

"*Miriam's Secret* provides an inspiring spark and fills an important void that nurtures the soul and garnishes our most personal journeys. This transformational work will warm your heart and nourish your mind's eye."
—**Joanne Loewy, DA, LCAT, MT-BC,** Director of the Louis Armstrong Music and Medicine Center, Beth Israel Hospital, and Associate Professor, Icahn School of Medicine, Mount Sinai

"Eliana Gilad is like an ancient priestess, bestowing enchantment and alchemy through rhythm and sound. She takes you to a very deep place and then lifts you to a beautiful high."
—**Marianne Williamson,** author of *A Return to Love* and *From Tears to Triumph*

your beautiful voices. Let them continue to be heard. They make a difference. ♥ Eliana

MIRIAM'S SECRET

REVEALING THE ANCIENT WISDOM OF FEMININE LEADERSHIP

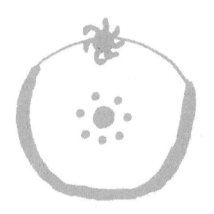

ELIANA GILAD

VOICES OF EDEN
GALILEE, ISRAEL

Eliana Gilad/Voices of Eden
HaGefen 20
Kiryat Tivon, Israel 36503
www.voicesofeden.com

Book Layout © 2017 BookDesignTemplates.com
Cover Design: Kit Foster and Victoria Davies (vikncharlie)
Cover photograph: Bella Shahar Hillel

Miriam's Secret – Revealing the Ancient Wisdom of Feminine Leadership/ Eliana Gilad. -- 1st ed.
ISBN 978-0-692-91613-1

This book is dedicated to all the feminine leaders
who dare listen to their inner voices and follow
their callings.
You are our true leaders.

CONTENTS

INTRODUCTION

Revealing the Ancient Wisdom of Feminine Leadership

Miriam's Secret is how to lead yourself through the unpredictable process of change. It's a soft, fluid, intuitive approach that helps you come full circle with your inner and outer conflicts so that you can live in harmony with yourself and others no matter what else is going on around you. By coming full circle, I mean that we tend to look outside ourselves for answers, when what we are truly looking is the clarity that resides deep within.

What's remarkable is that this powerful method of supporting yourself whenever you are going through a personal transformation of any kind comes from ancient sources that were lost to us for millennia. Today these sources are being rediscovered by archaeologists and through the rebirth of the intuitive dimension in our culture.

Perhaps this alternative way of nurturing, soothing, and leading yourself might work better than what you have been doing up until now. Or perhaps this approach might invite another means of connecting with your feminine power; like trusting that once you have done your best (at anything), believing that it is enough that *you* are enough. You rest, knowing that the results will occur, in their own time.

Miriam's Secret for managing change is a path of mindfulness. It is a means of deep inner listening, and of living in the now, present with whatever is. The good news is that this is a private experience, at its core both visceral and subjective. There is no right or wrong way to be mindful. You cannot screw it up or make a mistake.

Recovering the Lost Secret

The inspirational message of *Miriam's Secret* is that it helps you access your inner strength whether you're in the desert of facing life's challenges, persistently moving toward your goals, going through any kind of rebirth, or engaged in a process of growth. As you listen inwardly to yourself and draw sustenance from the well of wisdom inside, you are empowered to transform your life from the inside out, joyfully arriving at your personal Promised Land, however you define that.

Among the tools of the ancients that are being rediscovered and employed by contemporary healers and teachers, such as me, are simple, supportive, mindful, and healing sound techniques. Basically, these train you to show up and speak up. This ancient way of communing with yourself helps your nervous system to relax when it's being stimulated by the very thing that perturbs it. One simple, potent example is simply taking the time to listen to yourself while you're talking.

One reason the ancients understood the power of these tools and insights is that their world was different than ours. They were intimately connected to nature in a way most of us do not experience anymore —at least not in the developed nations of the Western world, where everything is mechanized and rigidly structured. Their connection to nature helped the ancients be more attuned to the fluid and shifting rhythms of life.

When we change our priorities and lifestyles to be more natural, and attune with our own inherent, creature rhythms, like they did, we gain greater access to, and appreciation for the power of the soft, flowing approach in our existence. Our lives become more balanced when we adopt principles such as "Less is more" and "Slow is the most direct route to the manifestation of anything." The quality of our self-connection improves when we do less and slow down, and this increases the quality of our connection with ourselves and others.

It feels vital for us to recover the wisdom of Miriam. There are so many changes going on in the world today—climatic changes, economic crises, wars, political unrest, to name only a few—that it seems kind of silly even to write about them. Media reports feature gloom and doom and the world coming to an end. But they don't tell us what happens next. They only inspire fear, which tends to be unproductive because it usually paralyzes us. In the feminine approach to life, destruction always brings the opportunity for rebirth. It's an opportunity for creation.

A rebirth of the soft flow is occurring in our culture right now, and a movement is forming: The challenges we face have driven us to reclaim the intuition. When everything is out of control and the old ways just don't work anymore, people feel vulnerable and unsafe. Spiritual leader Michael Beckwith calls this phenomenon a *birth-quake*. The feminine approach helps us to nurture ourselves in moments of birth-quake when we feel shaky.

Those who are willing to meet the process of cultural change openly are learning something wondrous about themselves and how they are connected to everyone and everything. This is good news. It was the impetus for me to begin writing this book.

Why Did I Write This Book?

I share Miriam's story with you as an act of service to the ancient way of feminine power. This is my contribution to the revival of the feminine voice of leadership. Many people are not familiar with Miriam the prophetess. Readers may think that they must have a religious background to relate to this material. Nothing could be further from the truth! Miriam's wisdom is rooted in a power that knows no division of race, creed, color, or religion.

You don't need to have any religious inclination to be able to relate to or gain from this material. Those who have been reared in a religious household will discover a new exploration from a different perspective than is usually shared. We will explore feminine leadership with its connection to the source of the universal power.

It is my hope that by acknowledging and exploring the spiritual authority of Miriam together, we will drink and be nourished by our collective well of wisdom.

The Impetus behind This Book

The impetus for this book came in the snow-covered mountains of the French Alps during the winter of 1992. I was working in the news research department of CBS television during the broadcasting of the Olympic Games from France. I was blessed with the job of broadcasting voiceovers for the opening and closing ceremonies, as well as doing preproduction vocals on a variety of lifestyle pieces to be broadcast during the Games.

The news research department is where decisions are made as to what to broadcast on the news. I sat next to a friendly gentleman whose job it was to read the wire services, such as the United Press, the Associated Press International, and Reuters, aiming to find newsworthy headlines that would be of interest for the daily news program.

Day after day, I would listen to his exclamatory "oohs" and "ahhs" in response to a headline. It drove me nuts, yet I had a difficult time reconciling whether to say something or keep my mouth shut. I wanted to speak my truth. I'm a feminine leader. Yet being able to stand in my power and express my voice without being shunned, attacked, or put down was a daily challenge for me back then.

Then, one day when he said, "Listen to this!" I interrupted him before he continued with, "I don't need to listen, because I already know what you are going to tell me."

"No, you don't," he replied.

"Yes, I do," I insisted.

"What?" he inquired.

"Don't you see?" I said, then continued, "It's always the same story of war, rape, pillage, murder, burglary, or disaster. Good news is a cease fire. Only the names and places change."

"That's not true. Let's look together," he said, challenging me. I moved my chair next to his so that we could watch the computer screen together. The situation was exactly as I had imagined. A sad joke began between us, as he promised, "I swear I'm going to find you your *good news* story." His intention was never fulfilled.

During those few months working for CBS, I silently prayed to the Divine to use my voice for a higher purpose. Little did I know then that my prayers would be answered less than a year later while singing on the inner-city trains of Paris. I did not know that my brief experience working within the world of mass media communications would spawn a new career for me that would lead to insights about drawing wisdom from our own inner wells. Although the experience with CBS was amazing, I still found myself working for a living. Inside me, a deep inner voice was drawing me to forth uncover my purpose in life.

When I decided to stop taking work just to pay the bills and to trust the wisdom inside me to guide me, not only did I discover that it is wise to listen to the inner voice, I learned that when we express it outwardly, it has a healing and transformational effect not only upon us, but also upon others. When people would ask me how I learned to produce the unique quality of vocal tones coming out of my mouth, their response to what I told them was frequently, "My God, that story sounds like a Hollywood movie. You have got to write down these anecdotes. Others will want to know about this."

Eventually, I had heard this response so many times, that I made a commitment that one day—when the time was right—I would follow through and write my stories down.

Writing this book is the culmination of that commitment I made twenty years ago singing on the trains, which is where I initially developed the Voices of Eden healing music approach that incorporates Miriam's Secret and the wisdom of the ancients living in the Near East. The story of how I got there is peppered throughout this book.

At this point, I was looking for my purpose in life. I had given up my mainstream, nine-to-five existence. Deep spiritual practice and implementing the inner tools of intuitive listening were my only daily guides. I had the good fortune of receiving tremendous support through colleagues in Los Angeles, such as Marianne Williamson, who had recently left a secretarial job and was risking her faith to give lectures about *A Course in Miracles*, Susan Jeffers who had just completed *Feel the Fear and Do It Anyway*, Jack Canfield, who back then was leading workshops in self-esteem within the elementary school system, and Barbara De Angelis, who was developing inspirational messages. Their support got me to take the leap I needed to leave the United States. We would meet at a weekly inspirational networking breakfast group called the Inside Edge, which provided us with practical support and camaraderie. It was through those meetings that I learned about a new technique called the Sedona Method and began to work with its creator, Lester Levenson, a man whom I consider to be one of the great gifts of my life.

Lester became my mentor. He taught me to stop looking outside of myself for answers when he would ask questions like: "How difficult could it be to be who you already are?" This provoked me into deep inner listening, which in today's lingo, would be called mindfulness. The release technique I learned from him would help me to release the habit of holding on. When Lester and I would meet, I would ask him for direction: What to do? How to proceed?

Lester's response was always, "Put your freedom first. Use the world to go free by. Make imperturbability, the state where no one or nothing can disturb your inner peace, your goal. Then have anything you will or desire."

His advice made sense to me. I made the decision to live by listening inside and being led by the gentle inner voice of wisdom which I found there.

If we dare follow the guidance of the inner voice, it will take us to good places. During an entire year, six days a week, I sang on the inner-city trains of Paris, which was my training ground (pun intended) for developing the ancient feminine healing sound and leadership model that I now teach. Call it a walking meditation or prayer. The process was always about showing up in the present moment, meeting the fear of death, or any other thought, feeling, or sensation that would come up in the moment. I never thought about what was coming out of my mouth. The words of the spirituals I sang served as the instruments through which I would release everything that arose to the contrary.

There was always something in my head that tried to stop me, thoughts like: *Are you nuts? You've gone crazy! What are you doing on this train? Stop this instant! What if your family saw you? What would they say!?* Fears and critical voices such as these were arising to keep me from showing up and following through on what that softer, deeper, oceanic voice within me was directing me to do. As I would release these resistant and frightened feelings one by one, a harmonious voice would just flow out of me. It was amazing grace. It amazed me then and it still does to this day.

During the entire year I spent singing on the trains, I never thought about the performance aspect of singing, nor was I doing it for money. I never once asked for money directly, and yet I received everything I needed to cover all my expenses from contributions people would hand to me spontaneously. The process was a sort of walking musical meditation, of showing up in each moment, naked like a newborn.

That year provided me with ample opportunity to discover the wisdom of feminine leadership, from the inside out, and to learn an alternative way of mindfully showing up for myself. It healed me of the tremendous shame of my father washing my mouth out with soap for speaking my truth, and ultimately it led to my moving to Israel to revive an ancient feminine sound healing and leadership technique. Over the years since then, this modality has been clinically researched and proven to lower blood pressure and heart rate, increase focus, and improve the quality of sleep.

My life experiences formed the basis of my personal transformation and self-connection, as well as establishing a foundation for my subsequent discoveries about the ancient healing and transformational knowledge discussed in this book. In *Miriam's Secret,* I am proposing a whole new idea of the Promised Land. Instead of it being a destination, the Promised Land is the powerful experience of self-connection or self-leadership. What if *you* are the destination you are searching for? It is simply about being you without changing a thing.

I invite you to explore Miriam's Secret with me and see if you do not find it as valuable in your own life as it has been in mine.

How to Use This Book

What began as one book, morphed into an entire series as an editor I worked with deftly pointed out to me that there were different trajectories in my material, paths related to leadership, healing music and sound, presentation, and my own personal story, each one powerful and meaty enough to warrant its own volume. The book you are holding in your hands today, is the first book in the series.

This book was published in the spring, the New Year of ancient times that coincides with the Passover holiday recounting the story of the Exodus from the Bible— including the parting of the waters of the Red Sea and freedom from slavery. When we use our voices like Miriam did, we have the power to lead ourselves through whatever we believe threatens to drown us and free ourselves from our personal bondage. This is a subjective experience that changes us inside and out. For when we change on the inside, the world around us responds—and we become more effective.

This book was written intuitively, through connection to the source of feminine power. Its organization arrived on the page through flow rather than by figuring it out intellectually. I therefore recommend that you contemplate and meditate upon this material. Its potency comes with repeated use

Each chapter in Part I of the book concludes with powerful questions designed to help you live from the heart of your feminine power, whether you are a woman or a man. They are designed to help you apply this material into your own life and support you in those areas where you may struggle to stand in your power and *be* yourself. Following the questions, I have provided additional space for you to respond.

Ancient Healing Music Meditation Bonus

Included with your purchase of *Miriam's Secret* are two gifts: a bonus music meditation MP3 and a Quick Start Action Guide PDF. Both can be downloaded from a special page on my website:

http://bit.ly/musicmiriam

Combining this dynamic music with the meditations you do in Part I of this book will increase your effectiveness in incorporating this feminine wisdom approach into your life. It will help you go deeper, faster.

There are four key aspects of the music that you should know.

- This ancient feminine healing music approach is medically researched and proven to increase focus and reduce stress.
- The music meditation was recorded live in ancient Israel.
- The music is 100 percent organic. There is no synthesized sound used. Everything you hear is real and natural.
- It is composed using an ancient feminine healing rhythm. It provides a container for those parts of us that are "off kilter" or "off balance." It allows space for those "untidy" parts of our being that we do not like. As you listen and allow space for these parts to speak

their truth to you, your greatest vulnerabilities may become your greatest strengths.

What You Will Discover in This Book
This book will address questions such as:

- Why do we listen to the critical voices inside us, letting them run us?
- Why are we so afraid of what others think of us?
- What if we put out something "bad"?
- How can we determine what we want out of life?

These are fundamental questions underlying our conscious thoughts. The answers require a different type of inquiry, one that is inner, rather than outer focused.

Miriam's world is a watery world. When you dive into her well, you will begin a journey that will lead you to your needed destination, even if you take the dive without knowing exactly where that destination is or how you will get there.

When you find yourself going through a major change or transition in your life, or you feel stuck somewhere, you can refer to this book. Let the mindfulness questions and the music meditation serve as your intimate companions.

There are three parts to this book. Part I of the book, "Connection," will help you reconnect to your own well of wisdom and can help you flow around the boulders that may be coming up as you move from one state of being to another. You will find exercises here.

Part II, "Courage," will help you gain courage from your inner well of wisdom, providing you with practical tools and a three-step process to cradle you on a fluid journey, one that is nurturing, nourishing, and supportive of the soft flow of life.

Part Three, "Confidence," will provide support in sharing your own song of wisdom within the world.

I hope that this book will become dog-eared, stained, and crumpled through repeated use. I hope that this will serve as an inspiration for you to gather in a circle with companions to collectively explore your own feminine leadership. In the process of working with this book, my hope is that you will realize you and your immediate companions are not alone.

Remember that the Promised Land is not an outcome; it is an experience of being at ease with who you are. This book will help you listen to yourself, and to drink from your own well of knowledge. When you live in this way, you can be in your Promised Land no matter what else may be going on around you. You will be nourished through your inner transformation, drinking from the sweet waters of life, and having more confidence being your true self.

If this promise resonates in your heart, then great, let's move on.

PART I
CONNECTION

Who was Miriam? While most people in the Western world have heard the story of the baby Moses being put in the bulrushes of the Nile River where he was rescued by the Pharaoh's daughter, fewer know the story of his older sister, Miriam, to whom he owes his life. The Bible reveals that by the time Miriam reached adulthood she had become a highly revered and respected prophetess among her people. When the ancient Hebrews fled from Egyptian oppression and safely crossed the Red Sea, she was with them. During their subsequent years of wandering through the desert looking for the Promised Land, it is said that Miriam had a magical well that appeared wherever she went that supplied water for their need.

Though there is not a lot written about Miriam in the Bible or in biblical commentary, what *is* written is significant. It proves that less is more. It shows how important it was for her to be included. If not, her story would have been erased altogether. When ideas or things are minimized, it shows their power by the very fact that their potency is being shunned to promote something different.

Each of the three Abrahamic faiths, Judaism, Christianity, and Islam, has its own version of a Miriam story. She is the representation of the feminine archetype.

CHAPTER 1

Miriam as Prophetess

Before Miriam's appearance in the Bible, she is described in Hebrew commentaries prophesying the birth of Moses. Egyptian Pharaoh Ramses II decreed that all male babies in Hebrew households were to be killed. In response, Amram, father of Miriam and the head of the Hebrew community, announced that he planned to divorce his wife so that they would not produce an infant the Pharaoh could kill. Miriam, only six years old at the time, says to her father:

> *Your decree is worse than Pharaoh. He decreed killing male babies. You separated from your wife and the entire community followed suit. Your behavior will cause our entire people to be destroyed. Take back your wife. She will give birth to a son, who will be the redeemer of our people.*
> —*Babylonian Talmud: Sotah 12b*

Amram listened to her and renounced the divorce. What Miriam declared came to pass and Moses was born. Who was the six-year-old who wielded this type of power? Obviously a known and respected leader, even at that age, for her father accepts and follows her direction.

Often children can see more than their parents. I myself was born with a high level of clarity. I remember being six years old and observing the interaction between my father, mother, and older brother as if I were watching a play. The role each one was playing in our family drama was crystal clear. As I grew up, I learned to play my part as well, yet it was important for me to stay connected to the source of my true power. Not that it was always easy.

We are all born leaders. Each one of us has a special role to play. Contrasting experiences allow us to develop our inner resources.

In the Hebrew Bible, the Torah, it is written that Miriam was the older sister of Moses and Aaron. She is the only woman to be named a prophetess in her own right.

Here are some questions for you to ponder that may help to revive your own sense of feminine leadership.

• What leadership qualities did you exhibit as a child?

_____

_____

_____

_____

_____

_____

_____

_____

_____

_____

_____

_____

• Where do you see children having leadership qualities that you could nurture?

_____

_____

_____

_____

_____

_____

_____

_____

_____

_____

_____

_____

_____

_____

_____

- How could you nurture those same qualities within yourself?

_____

_____

_____

_____

_____

_____

_____

_____

_____

_____

_____

CHAPTER 2

Miriam as Protector

In Exodus 2, Miriam—although she is not named—is described as standing on the riverbank watching over her brother, Moses. Pharaoh's decree of death to all Hebrew boys was still in effect, so shortly after Moses' birth, his mother, Yocheved, set him adrift in a basket in the river. Miriam watched over him from the bulrushes and protected him from harm. She saw to it that Pharaoh's daughter found the baby and took him in. Miriam also saw to it that their mother, Yocheved, served as Moses' wet nurse in the palace.

Then said his [Moses'] sister to Pharaoh's daughter, "Shall I go and call to thee a nurse of the Hebrew women that she may nurse the child for you? And Pharaoh's daughter said to her, "Go." And the maid went and called the child's mother. And Pharaoh's daughter said to her, "Take this child away, and nurse it for me, and I will give you your wages." And the woman [Yocheved] took the child [Moses, her baby] and nursed it.
—Numbers 2

Miriam saw to it that her mother—also Moses' mother—would earn money to nurse her own son. No one stood in her way. Given the power she wielded in negotiating for Pharaoh's daughter to take Moses, her brother, into the palace, it's not much of a stretch to imagine that Miriam would have had the Pharaoh's daughter's ear. She likely may have had direct connection to Pharaoh as well.

Deep inside, we do know our places in the world. Even though we may not be able to articulate them with specific words, an inner sense of knowing will whisper the truth in our ears if we are willing to listen.

In 1994, I was living in France, at a crossroads and wondering what was next for me, I planned a trip to Israel with a friend of mine who dreamed of pilgrimage to the Holy Land for her birthday during the Passover-Easter season. A few days before our trip, she suddenly disappeared from my life without a trace. I was left alone to travel on my nonrefundable airplane ticket. After the shock, I realized this was evidently an opportunity for me to experience my personal parting of the seas.

The voice in me whispered: "Move to Israel, settle in Galilee where you will establish a center in a green place where one sees blue, where there will be special music that combines East and West, computers with a focus over the seas." I had no idea what that meant. Yet after so many experiences of listening to that small still voice inside, I knew to pay attention. I packed my bags and soon moved to Israel.

- How can Miriam's role as protector help empower you in your life?

_____

_____

_____

_____

_____

_____

_____

_____

_____

_____

_____

CHAPTER 3

Miriam as Priestess

From history, we can imagine that Miriam was raised to serve as a midwife and temple priestess for a female deity, one with specialized knowledge of sacred healing practices, among them toning, drumming, and meditation. I believe Miriam was a priestess in the cult of Hathor, an Egyptian deity ruling healing, music, and childbirth. It would make sense: The presence and influence of women's cults in early Israel is a well-known fact. Archaeological finds, as well as multiple books written on the subject, such as *Did God Have a Wife?* by William Dever and *The Hebrew Goddess* by Raphael Patai, document this subject at length.

It is easy to see this influence in the story of Exodus by looking at the Egyptian goddess Hathor that Alison Roberts writes about so eloquently in her book *Hathor Rising*. Hathor's son, Ihy, is represented as a golden calf, which helps in the difficult birth and change. As Roberts describes, Ihy is like "the animal whose tracks are followed by travelers in difficult desert terrain—indeed a guide for those in the difficult passage of new birth."

Later, after the division of the tribes of Israel into two kingdoms, Israel and Judah, King Jeroboam of Israel set up two golden calf idols, one at Dan and the other at Bethel, in an attempt to keep the people of the northern kingdom of Israel from going to Jerusalem, and in the southern kingdom of Judah, to worship. Jeroboam referred to his calf idols in the same words that Aaron used centuries before, as "your gods, O Israel, who brought you up out of the land of Egypt."

The king took counsel, and made two calves of gold. And he said to the people, "You have gone up to Jerusalem long enough. Behold your gods, O Israel, who brought you up out of the land of Egypt"" And he set one in Bethel, and the other he put in Dan. And this thing became a sin, for the people went to the one at Bethel and to the other as far as Dan.
—1 Kings 12:26–30

What if Ihy, Hathor's son, were the golden calf to whom the Israelites worshipped in the desert when Moses went up Mount Sinai to receive the Ten Commandments, and later in the sanctuaries of Dan and Bethel?

The priestesses of Hathor were the mentors, obstetricians, psychologists, and healers of their time. In the temple of Hathor in Egypt, music was used for healing and transformational purposes, and protection for safe birth. The ancients understood and had deep knowledge of the conscious use of voice and rhythm as a natural healing technology. Sound vibration was the medium that they employed to manage change and attune to harmonious living. The need to access intuition, wisdom, and creativity as a means of "attunement" was essential to safely conceive, create, and usher in new lives. It was a fundamental aspect in the ancient way of feminine leadership.

A recent archaeological exhibition at the Oriental Institute of the University of Chicago explored the life of a temple singer named Meresamun dating from 800 B.C.E. The name Meresamun in ancient Egyptian means "beloved of Amun," who was the sun god. Meresamun lived in Ancient Thebes. In her coffin were seventy objects, an archeological find that provides a vivid idea of her lifestyle.

The brief inscription on Meresamun's coffin states that she was a "singer in the interior of the Temple of Amun at Karnak." She, along with other women from elite families, served in the temple, playing music for the god as the priests laid offerings and purifications before the deity. We know from other sources that singers like Meresamun were probably trained by their mothers, and often several generations of women from a single family worked as temple singers.

In Meresamun's era, women held the post of singer inside the temple, although men played instruments in rituals held outside the temple. Her title, Singer in the Interior of the Temple, indicates that she had a level of purity that allowed her to enter the most sacred part of the divine complex.

I find it interesting that this title so closely relates to the description of the Levite priests entering the sacred part of temple. Aaron, Miriam's brother, is known as the first Hebrew priest. The reference of music in the temple refers to the Levites being the ones who would play in service to the Divine. In both cases, we can see that music was consciously used and practiced in Hebrew worship.

Here are two questions for you to ponder.

- How can remembering the past help you in your present life?

_____

_____

_____

_____

_____

_____

_____

_____

_____

_____

_____

_____

_____

_____

_____

_____

_____

_____

_____

- How might learning about forgotten cultures and reconnecting the pieces of the puzzle from ancient cultures help us in our modern lives today?

_____

_____

_____

_____

_____

_____

_____

CHAPTER 4
Miriam as Midwife

Rabbinical scholars identify Miriam with Puah, one of the two Hebrew midwives, Shiphrah and Puah, who served the Israelites during the Egyptian enslavement. These two midwives are credited with refusing to follow Pharaoh's decree of death for male Hebrew babies—a clear act of civil disobedience. The scholars differ on whether Yocheved was Shiprah and Miriam was Puah.

The name Puah embodies two different character traits in Miriam's personality: On the one hand, she shows sensitivity and tenderness; on the other, she acts assertively and aggressively both to her father and to Pharaoh. These dual characteristics are common traits of feminine deities of ancient times, such as Sekhmet-Hathor in ancient Egypt, Inanna-Ereshkegal in the

Assyrian pantheon, and Asherah-Anat in the ancient
Hebrew tradition.

There is also a connection with the Kosharot described by scholars as the sacred Hebrew patronesses
of childbirth. Consider these deities as the ancient Israel roots of the classical Greek Charities or Graces,
embodiments of beauty, charm, and creativity, which
were known all over the ancient Near East and Medi-
terranean regions.

Feminine leadership qualities are different than
masculine leadership qualities in that they include not
only action-oriented directives, but also the ever-im-
portant intuitive side. Intuition includes the emotional
side of existence. When you're going through a period
of change and you don't know which way to go, which
choice to make, or there is no precedent for the change
you're going through, it's more important to feel your
way through things rather than figure them out. In the
process of "feeling things out" there may be a tug of war
between our rational sides and our intuitive sides.

Here are two questions to ponder related to this
topic.

- How can the role of a midwife help guide us into a
  new model of leading life today?

  _____

  _____

  _____

  _____

_____

_____

_____

_____

_____

_____

_____

_____

_____

_____

_____

_____

_____

_____

_____

- How could allowing space for the murky sides of life help you move to a new level of personal power?

_____

_____

_____

_____

_____

_____

_____

_____

_____

_____

_____

_____

_____

_____

_____

_____

_____

_____

_____

_____

_____

_____

_____

_____

_____

_____

_____

_____

_____

_____

_____

_____

CHAPTER 5

Miriam as Healing Musician

Miriam would have known how to employ meditation, sound, and rhythm in advanced ways. We know from the remains of Middle Eastern temples that those skills were respected by the people in the type of community she served. It wasn't just the prophetess Miriam who held this knowledge. All women in the temples of her era in history would have had it.

Archaeologists have uncovered clues about the activities of ancient sacred sisterhoods of prebiblical times. As a prophetess, a spiritual leader and wisdom mentor for her community, Miriam would have taught her people the secrets of taking the inward journey, using methods that included song, rhythm, vibration, and pace.

The Hebrews who escaped from Egypt would have followed these more ancient ways once Israel was reached. The musical customs and practices of the Levite priests in the main temple that was founded in Jerusalem (which still exists today, although all but its western wall is buried underground) similarly reflect the feminine music practices of prebiblical times.

With Miriam leading the way, sacred practices would have accompanied the Hebrew refugees from the "old country" to the "new."

Here are two questions to ponder.

•   How does your body respond to the ancient rhythm?

_____

_____

_____

_____

_____

_____

_____

_____

_____

_____

_____

_____

_____

_____

_____

_____

_____

_____

_____

_____

_____

_____

_____

_____

_____

_____

- How could you use healing sound into your day to help you connect to the source of your inner wisdom?

_____

_____

_____

_____

_____

_____

_____

_____

_____

_____

CHAPTER 6

Miriam as Leader

According to both written and oral scriptures, the Israelites viewed Miriam as one of the three central figures leading the people during the Exodus from Egypt and the march through the wilderness.

> *In fact, I brought you up from the land of Egypt, I redeemed you from the house of bondage. And I sent before you Moses, Aaron, and Miriam"*
> —Micah 6:4

> *Israel had three fine leaders, namely: Moses, Aaron, and Miriam.*
> —Ta'anit 9a

Miriam is portrayed in the sources mentioned above as a powerful prophetess who cares for Israel's needs in the wilderness. In the Sifre Deuteronomy 275, we see that she was a leader of leaders and of all tribes in the wilderness. The commentary tells of the Israelite camps setting out with only Miriam in their lead.

- How do you see feminine leadership?

_____

_____

_____

_____

_____

_____

_____

_____

_____

_____

_____

_____

_____

_____

_____

_____

_____

_____

_____

_____

_____

_____

_____

_____

_____

- How can feminine traits of leadership, help care for our needs in the "wilderness" of modern life?

_____

_____

_____

_____

_____

_____

_____

_____

_____

_____

_____

_____

_____

_____

_____

CHAPTER 7

Miriam as Mentor

Miriam acted as a mentor to Moses. Since Miriam was his elder sister and accepted as a powerful prophetess he would most likely have turned to her for advice. There is early precedence of Miriam prophesizing his birth, and of their father recognizing her power and following her advice. Moses, as the younger child, would have followed this lead.

Miriam's feminine leadership was instrumental from the start. Given that she would have had the ear of Pharaoh's daughter and likely that of Pharaoh himself, it is easy to imagine how Moses would have been mentored by Miriam to speak and stand up to authority. Her power that was so instrumental in arranging for Moses to be taken into the royal house would be extremely useful to help free their people from slavery.

Miriam and her well provided the people with nurturance during their transformation from a weary group of slaves to an empowered group of free men and women.

Here is a question to consider.

- Who has been an instrumental mentor in your life? What qualities did this individual exhibit that created such an important impact upon you?

_____

_____

_____

_____

_____

_____

_____

_____

_____

_____

_____

_____

_____

CHAPTER 8

Miriam and the Song at the Sea

Miriam is first mentioned by name in a passage in a section of the Bible known as the Song at the Sea.

> *Then Miriam the prophetess, Aaron's sister, took a drum in her hand, and all the women went out after her in dance with drums. And Miriam chanted for them, "Sing to the Lord, for He has triumphed gloriously; horse and driver He has hurled into the sea."*
> *—Exodus 15:20–21*

The former Hebrew slaves have crossed over the parted seas. The waters have miraculously crashed down upon the Egyptian soldiers that were pursuing them. Miriam sings out in praise, expressing what most would be thinking and may not have dared to express. She was centered and secure in her power, and that voice and rhythm were the established means of communicating it. This biblical passage is one of the best proofs of ancient feminine wisdom leadership.

Here are a couple of questions for you to consider.

• What would you truly like to express that others around you are thinking, but dare not say out loud?

_____

_____

_____

_____

_____

_____

_____

_____

_____

_____

_____

_____

_____

_____

_____

_____

_____

_____

_____

_____

_____

_____

_____

_____

_____

_____

_____

_____

_____

- How might expressing this increase your personal sense of power and leadership?

_____

_____

_____

_____

_____

_____

_____

_____

_____

_____

_____

_____

CHAPTER 9

Miriam Speaks Against Moses

Miriam appears in the biblical book of Numbers, when she and her brother Aaron speak against the Cushite wife of Moses. They state that God has spoken to them, too, implying their discontent with the shift in status quo between themselves and their younger brother. Once again, Miriam shows her confidence in her leadership role through her behavior. Although both Aaron and Miriam are upset, it is Miriam who voices her discontent out loud. She is stricken with leprosy as punishment for speaking up.

Upon seeing Miriam's punishment, Aaron asks Moses to speak to God on her behalf. Moses responds immediately, crying out: "O Lord, please heal her." Though she acted defiantly, Miriam's powerful status in the eyes of her entire people is irrefutable.

> *Miriam was shut out of camp seven days; and the people did not march on until Miriam was readmitted.*
> —*Numbers 12:15*

The scriptures show that the Hebrews were loyal to their leader, Miriam. They would not advance through the desert until she could continue with them. God eventually heals Miriam. The people wait. When she returns, the community moves on.

True leaders inspire courage, patience, and devotion in their followers. Even when facing controversy and challenge, a powerful leader will inspire others to act for the highest good.

Here are three questions to ponder.

- What leadership quality could you develop that would inspire courage, patience, and devotion in you and in others to things that will be important accomplishments?

_____

_____

_____

_____

_____

_____

_____

_____

_____

_____

_____

_____

- How could those qualities inspire you when you are
  facing a controversy or a challenge?

_____

_____

_____

_____

_____

_____

_____

_____

_____

_____

_____

_____

_____

- How would these same qualities inspire others?

_____

_____

_____

_____

_____

_____

_____

_____

_____

_____

_____

_____

_____

_____

_____

_____

_____

_____

_____

_____

CHAPTER 10

Miriam's Death

In different Jewish scriptures and rabbinical commentaries, we learn that, like her brothers, Moses and Aaron, Miriam died at Mount Nebo, a mountain overlooking the Promised Land. According to rabbinic commentary, the Angel of Death had no power over Miriam and she died by a kiss from God, a death that tradition holds is reserved for the "righteous." Apparently, worms were unable to consume Miriam. Mystically, Miriam was at such a high level that she was unaffected by the physical laws of the universe. In our modern era, this is like the exalted spiritual state that certain yogis reach, such as Paramahansa Yogananda, who it is said consciously left his body at the end of his life.

I suspect that Miriam had such a high level of consciousness that she was beyond identifying herself with her physical body. As a powerful prophetess who was schooled in the power of sound and rhythm to move matter, she would have had the power to leave her body at will.

Here are two questions for your consideration.

- Have you ever experienced sound, rhythm, or music in such a profound way that it moved worlds within you?

_____

_____

_____

_____

_____

_____

_____

_____

_____

_____

_____

_____

_____

_____

_____

_____

_____

_____

_____

_____

_____

_____

- What was the experience like for you?

_____

_____

_____

_____

_____

_____

_____

_____

_____

_____

_____

_____

_____

_____

_____

_____

CHAPTER 11

Miriam's Well

The main function of wells is to provide a source of drinking water for humans and their animals. Rain, springs, and brooks are natural sources of water. Wells are an invention of human knowledge and skill that arose with the invention of tools strong enough to penetrate deeply into earth or rock to reach water hidden underground.

Wells in the Bible are also referred to as meeting places. In an article entitled "Wells, Women and Faith," Joan Cook traces a recurring pattern found in biblical sources: (1) A man journeys to a foreign land; (2) he encounters a woman or women; (3) someone draws water; (4) a woman runs home to announce the visitor's arrival; (5) the visitor is invited to a meal.

During the Israelites' journey through the desert toward the Promised Land, anticipation of getting to a water source brought forth a song of joy. This is the song of the well at which the Divine spoke to Moses:

> *Assemble the people that I may give them water.*
> *—Numbers 21:16*

> *Spring up, O well*
> *Sing to it*
> *The well which the chieftains dug,*
> *Which the nobles of the people started*
> *With maces, with their own staffs.*
> *—Numbers 21:17–18*

The story of Miriam's death in Numbers 20 is immediately followed by the story of the waters of Meribah. This story recounts how the community was without water. When Miriam dies, the result is drought; the well that accompanied the Israelites in the wilderness and provided them with drinking water dries up. The well, according to biblical commentary, was one of the things created at twilight on Sabbath eve.

Later tradition tells that when Miriam died, angels hid her well along the shores of Galilee.

Miriam's well can be understood as providing both physical sustenance as well as emotional and spiritual nourishment during her people's time of wandering. Her nurturance kept them afloat during the most perilous and difficult of journeys. Her spiritual leadership helped people believe in a power greater than themselves who would always come through.

Here are two questions to reflect upon.

- What helps you believe in a power greater than yourself that you can turn to in times of need?

_____
_____
_____
_____
_____
_____
_____
_____
_____
_____
_____
_____
_____
_____
_____
_____

- Where do you go to receive a well of inspiration?

_____

_____

_____

_____

_____

_____

_____

_____

_____

_____

_____

_____

_____

_____

_____

_____

_____

_____

_____

_____

_____

_____

PART II
COURAGE

The prophetess Miriam was Divine Feminine power incarnate when she was leading people through perilous times toward their Promised Land. By exploring the story of Miriam, we reclaim lost parts of ourselves that we forgot long ago. This brings joy back into our lives and enables us to serve as positive examples for others who are looking to live with more meaning.

In Part II, we will dig more deeply to explore what Miriam's life means to us during our modern times of tumultuous change. You'll discover that you are so much more courageous than you think you are. Miriam teaches us to respect and appreciate those parts of ourselves that we cannot see. Then we will look at how you can apply these teachings on your own journey toward your personal Promised Land.

CHAPTER 12

Miriam and Sacred Traditions

When the structures of convention have broken down, people are left to fend for themselves. In a world where self-esteem and worth are often built upon how much we achieve, many of us find ourselves working harder now for fewer rewards. The old systems of our world no longer work. We are living in a time where almost anything goes. If you're used to following your own path, this may seem like great news. If you were happy with the status quo, it could be terrifying.

Miriam's story is more relevant today than ever before. The prophetess was rooted in her power. She needed no outside confirmation of her value or decision-making abilities. She needed no convention. She spoke her truth and she acted according to it. Miriam is an excellent model of authentic power, which cannot be contained by outer forces.

Let's examine how Miriam's story and the demonstration of her power are relevant to us.

CHAPTER 13

What Is Feminine Leadership?

Feminine-style leadership is visceral. It is intuitive. Decisions are made by inner knowing. Once all the details have been considered, the leader meditates and listens inwardly for direction. Then the leader remains open to receive an answer. It may take time. This requires patience. But it's worth the wait, as inner wisdom rarely fails us. Perhaps this explains why it is so scary to the masculine-dominated ego, which likes to be in control and to understand what is going on. With feminine leadership, many layers of reality are accommodated at the same time. It may not make sense.

Being a seer and keeper of wisdom, Miriam was adept at ensuring that ancient traditions would be kept alive. Miriam used her leadership to protect these ways and carry them forward. By going undercover and weaving them into the evolving masculine worldview, she preserved and sheltered feminine knowledge until the world would be ready for it to reemerge into the light. She saw the transformation of her culture occurring. Instead of preparing for conflict and making war, she surrendered to flow with the tides of change. This is the mark of a true leader. It is a beautiful expression of feminine power. A shift is reoccurring once again today.

CHAPTER 14

The Divine Feminine Principle and Miriam

Miriam is an important archetypal representation of the Divine Feminine. Even her name in Hebrew is feminine. It flows with the music of water, which alludes to her oceanic power.

Miriam מרים-

Mem (מ), the first letter of her name in Hebrew, means "from," as in "from the inside out." The circular shape of the letter mem symbolizes a womb space. All

around the globe, the sound "M" represents both creation and the mother. The word for mother, in most
languages around the world, contains the sound of the
letter "M": *mama, maman, amma,* and *mommy,*
for example.

Resh (ר), the next letter in Miriam's name, in ancient
times symbolized the sound of fire. Ra was the name of
the Egyptian Sun god, ruler of the light. Creation came
from light. We see its transformation in the Bible in
Genesis 1:3. "And God said: 'Let there be Light.'"

Yam (ים), which is the combined sound of the next
two letters in Miriam's name, means "ocean." In addi-
tion, the Hebrew word for water, *mayim,* is contained
in Miriam's name. As is *rim,* which means to "raise up,"
and *ram,* which means "grand."

CHAPTER 15

Miriam as an Archetypal Symbol of the Divine Mother

Conventional explanations of Miriam's name define its meaning as "bitter sea" or "bitter water," because *mem* and *resh* combined represent the word *bitter*. I see things from another perspective, without bitterness. I view Miriam as the archetypal symbol of divine mothering power, a blessing. She represents an oceanic womb of power, whose unpredictability produces the birth of light, the sun, and all of creation.

The waters of the womb are dark, and pregnancy is an emotional passage for a mother. Perhaps this is the aspect of Miriam's name to which "bitter" refers. Yet a baby in the womb is also nourished and sustained by amniotic fluid, the mother's "waters."

The word for well in Hebrew is *maayan* (מעין). The first letter of this word is *mem*, the same as the first letter of Miriam's name, which, as you'll recall, means "from," as in "from the inside out." The form of the letter reflects this as well. It is round and cylindrical, has an opening, and flows energetically from within, through the bottom up rather than from the head down.

The rest of the word is composed of the three letters that spell the Hebrew word *ayin* (עין), which means "eye," as in to "see."

CHAPTER 16

Sekhmet—Hathor—Miriam— Mother Mary

The ancient feminine archetype of visceral, intuitive power is the leonine goddess Sekhmet, who was known as the "Mother of All." She held the entire cosmos at her command. Her raw power was so great that she was venerated and greatly feared as well. Centuries later, her feline ferociousness transformed into the cow goddess Hathor, who was associated with love and healing.

With her knowledge of the cult of Hathor, the prophetess Miriam would likely have been connected to the powers of Sekhmet as well. Since Sekhmet held the power to create and destroy entire universes, this might explain the power of Miriam's voice and rhythm as a force that could have parted the waters of the Red Sea, allowing for the Israelites to safely cross it.

It is understood by the Sophian Gnostics that Miriam reincarnated as Mother Mary. Mary's name in Hebrew is Miriam. Like the prophetess Miriam, Mary is represented as divine female energy. Mother Mary/prophetess Miriam are the nurturing, matriarchal forces that guide humanity through the trials and tribulations of life.

CHAPTER 17

The Rise of the Feminine

It is telling that so powerful a figure as Miriam is scarcely mentioned in the scriptures that have been handed down to us. This points to a diminishment of her importance for a reason. I believe this was done to show the rise of Moses' leadership as a cognitive worldview took precedence over a visceral one.

Seasons come and seasons go, and there are cycles to human history as well.

The world is really changing now. Today, the feminine is on the rise once again. This is a very constructive development. We can see it being expressed through the communal, inclusive design of modern office spaces. Today they are designed to support greater collaboration and relationship building, which are feminine qualities. Neuroscience and social science are also pointing to the value of diversity in managing the complexity of cataclysmic change.

The collaborative approach is feminine by nature. Just look at the worldwide web for collaborative approaches to communication, which is essential to leading in complex environments during complex times. Mindfulness in the workplace is on the rise, providing workers with the ability to connect within during their otherwise hectic schedules.

While it's easy to see imbalance in the world, it's heartening to contemplate the quiet shift of seismic proportions occurring beneath our feet. This is a time for rebalance.

Miriam's voice is being rebirthed. I believe it is an important step to restoring harmony to humanity.

CHAPTER 18

The Dual Nature of Feminine Power

All of us have dark and light sides to our personalities. In ancient times, these were expressed culturally through the worship of goddesses with dual natures. In the Middle East, the goddess Anat was known as the Storm God. Look at any major archaeological excavation in the region, and you'll find her presence there in one form or another. The most prevalent worship of her occurred from the Middle Bronze Age (2000–1500 B.C.E.) to the early Iron Age (900–600 C.E.). Ugaritic mythology, from the region of modern-day northern

Syria, which closely resembles Hebrew mythology, describes Anat as spending most of her time on the battlefield. Legend says that she was bloodthirsty and could be easily provoked to violence. Once she began to fight, she'd go berserk, smiting and killing. The stories describe her as fighting with real pleasure.

On the motherly side, despite her immense bloodlust, Anat was said to have been one of the wet nurses of the gods. The stories of Anat share commonality with the story of Sekhmet, who after storming and smiting, would be transformed into the mother goddess Hathor.

According to the *New World Encyclopedia,* the imagery of Anat appears prominently in Ancient Egyptian, Mesopotamian, and Hebrew cultures. She is represented as follows.

Anat in Egypt (Entry from the *New World Encyclopedia*)

"Anat first appears in Egypt in the sixteenth dynasty (the Hyksos period) along with other northwest Semitic deities. She was especially worshiped here in her aspect of a war goddess, often paired with the goddess Ashtarte, whose role was more strictly that of fertility. In the *Contest Between Horus and Set,* these two goddesses appear as daughters of Re and are given in marriage to Set, who may have been identified with the Semitic god Baal-Hadad.

"During the Hyksos period, Anat had temples in the Hyksos capital of Tanis (Egypt) and in Beth-Shan (Palestine), as well as being worshiped in Memphis. On inscriptions from Memphis of fifteenth to twelfth centuries B.C.E., Anat is called 'Bint-Ptah,' Daughter of Ptah. She is associated with Reshpu, (*Canaanite*: Resheph) in some texts and sometimes identified with the native Egyptian goddess Neith. She is sometimes called 'Queen of Heaven.' Her iconography varies, but she is usually shown carrying one or more weapons....

"In the Hebrew Bible, the wife of the patriarch Joseph, was named Senath, which may mean 'holy to Anath.' She is described as having been given to him by an unnamed Pharaoh who also gave Joseph the Egyptian name Zaphenath-Paneah."

Anat in Mesopotamia (Entry from the *New World Encyclopedia*)

"Antu or Antum is a Babylonian goddess, and seems to be a precursor of the Semitic Anat. She was the first consort of Anu, and the pair were the parents of the Anunnaki and the Utukki. Antu was an important feature in some Babylonian festivals until as recently as 200 B.C.E., but in general was replaced as Anu's consort by Ishtar/Inanna. . . . . .

"It has also been suggested just as the Sumerian goddess Inanna is related to her West Semitic counterpart, Ishtar, so in Canaanite tradition the two goddesses Anath and Astarte are closely linked, particularly in the poetry of Ugarit. In iconography, it is often difficult for archaeologists to assign a name to a female deity holding a weapon or sheaf of grain, since such a description could apply to any of the above."

Anat in Israel (Entry from the *New World Encyclopedia*)

"The goddess Anat is not mentioned in Hebrew scriptures as a goddess per se. However, it is possible that she may be confused with the goddesses Asherah and Astarte in the minds of the biblical writers. The term *asherim* is used frequently in the Bible to refer to sacred pillars erected by Canaanites and Israelites alike, in association with altars devoted to both Baal and Yahweh.

"Nevertheless, Anat's influence on Israelite culture was significant. Joseph's Egyptian wife, Asenath, named in honor of Anat, is traditionally believed to be the mother of Ephraim and Manasseh, and thus the foremother of these important Israelite tribes as well.

"The Israelite judge Shamgar 'son of Anath' is mentioned in Judges 3:31; 5:6, which raises the idea that this hero may have been imagined as a demigod, a mortal son of the goddess. However, John Day, in his book *Yahweh and the Gods and Goddesses of Canaan* (Sheffield Academic Press, 2000), notes that a number of Canaanites known from nonbiblical sources bore that title and theorizes that it was a military designation indicating a warrior under Anat's protection.

"Anat's name is preserved in the city names Beth Anath and Anathoth, the latter being the hometown of the prophet Jeremiah. Jeremiah uses one of Anat's titles in his prophecies against goddess-worship:

> *The children gather wood, the fathers light the fire, and the women knead the dough and make cakes of bread for the Queen of Heaven. They pour out drink offerings to other gods to provoke me to anger.*
> —Jeremiah 7:18, see also 44:17–19

"In Elephantine (modern Aswan) in Egypt, Jewish mercenaries, c. 410 B.C.E., left documents that make mention of a goddess called Anat-Yahu (Anat-Yahweh) worshiped in the local temple of Yahweh, originally built by Jewish refugees from the Babylonian conquest of Judah."

Shadows Transform Vulnerability into Strength

Whether represented within the Ancient Egyptian, Mesopotamian, or Israelite cultures, across them all, Anat clearly represented the shadow side of our feminine nature. When the shadow part of us gets shut off, in my experience we self-destruct. But when we meet those dark parts with compassion, we can midwife the motherly sides of ourselves. We become our own wet-nurses, who suckle the divine side of our natures.

Before I understood the motherly component of the fierce Anat archetype, I used to believe that if I'd get it "just right," I'd accomplish what my inner guidance was guiding me to do. I would drive myself so hard that I would collapse from exhaustion. With this single-minded focus to "accomplish and achieve" I put my relationships with myself and others at risk.

How? My definition of success was what I "achieved" . . . what I had "accomplished" . . . today . . . and tomorrow (as if that was possible!)! This motivated me to "do" a lot, yet there'd always be one more thing to do, and one more thing, and one more . . . causing me to have a feeling of "never enough."

All the seemingly great stuff being done, ignored my need just to *be*. It cut me off from who I AM. It was also a clever way to avoid the dark underbelly of my untidy vulnerability that threatened to blow my "super doer" cover. By not creating space for the untidy truth, I was denying my softness, my allowing, and my ability to receive.

In essence, I was "doing" a lot, but not really achieving much.

Our sense of openness and vulnerability allows us to connect and collaborate with others. Yet we can't do that without owning our shadow side. We need to be in touch with both sides of our nature. This is what provides us with balance.

The ancient wisdom of feminine leadership is that it cherishes both sides—light and dark—and holds them both as sacred. This wisdom is important for us to embrace today, as the conventional masculine ways of being no longer are serving us well in our complex culture.

To step into a new paradigm of feminine leadership—one that prioritizes ease, abundance, and grace—we must learn to accept *the shadow side of ourselves* that inadvertently shows up in ways that don't serve our highest good.

By acknowledging and accepting the untidy shadow side, it can become one of our biggest gifts.

The way of wisdom is a balance between deep inner listening and trusting your inner voice. From there, you can reach out and share what it is the voice is guiding you to contribute. While it can feel scary to express your tender, vulnerable side, it is also courageous. When feeling the fear and going ahead anyway, you transform your negatives into positives and develop true self-esteem and authentic power.

CHAPTER 19

What Was Miriam's Role in History?

Miriam's role was to lead humanity through an epic period of catalytic change. Miriam could say what no one else could say. We, as a civilization, were moving from a feminine-based worldview of nomadic tribalism to a masculine-based worldview of settlement. From feeling to analysis. Some scholars believe that as civilization made a shift from pictographic writing styles, such as hieroglyphics, to linear writing styles, such as the alphabet, it altered how our brains work. We lost contact with important ways of perceiving and sensing that had been very effective for us.

Going Beyond Understanding to Knowing

The Hebrew Bible demonstrates the shift from a worldview that was visceral and experiential to an intellectual approach that favored reasoning. In modern life, our attitude toward change and transformation is to regard that which is new as superior and more advanced than that which preceded it. We tend to reject tradition in favor of technology.

Understanding comes from the mind. It's an intellectual experience. You can read it in a book. This is a masculine attribute.

Knowing, by contrast, is a direct experience. When you know something, *you* are the book. This is a feminine attribute.

CHAPTER 20

Wells and Water Share a Feminine Quality

Miriam's Secret is that we have our own well of wisdom within us. We have a direct line to the Source of the entire power of the universe, if we will only stop long enough to connect with it, and if necessary, do the work of digging down, no matter what gets stirred up. We connect to wisdom's flow by slowing down.

Miriam's well represents the deep knowledge of this direct power. It is intuitive knowledge that is only gained by stopping and listening within. You arrive at knowing by being willing to dive beneath the shallow surface of your thoughts, soiling your hands in the silt and mud as you dig your way down to the sweet water of deep wisdom.

For thousands of years, people have relied on wells to thrive in even the harshest desert conditions. The ancients knew to dig down, scooping out sand and mud to reach clean water deep below the Earth's surface. There, the cool waters flow. Going from understanding to knowing is a similar process.

Water is powerful and virtually unstoppable. Water amplifies sound four times more powerfully than air. Drip water one drop at a time over a long period in the same spot and it can penetrate even the hardest rock. Throw a small pebble into a lake and the ripple effect it creates will form countless waves that grow out of that one small action.

Wells are ancient symbols of nourishment and nurturance. They also provide physical sustenance for life. This is particularly important to people living in arid deserts. The well was the meeting place where important encounters and contracts would be made. Mystically, wells also represent the divine feminine womb space, the source of life and creativity.

Silent acts of caring and love, these are the special gifts that feminine energy provides humanity. When we shut feminine qualities out of our lives, we "throw the baby out with the bathwater." Which is not unlike Moses floating in the bulrushes.

Without the ripple effect of Miriam's action to save Moses, no one would have been able to listen to the words of Moses. If not for Miriam's presence, he would not have been saved. Similarly, if we do not listen to our own soft and silent presence deep within, then we can never express the fullness of our authentic gifts.

But how is it possible to listen to this presence when life today is filled with so much chaos and static noise?

CHAPTER 21

Birth and Water as Signs of Transformation

The process of birth is one of the best examples of the chrysalis effect, or shifting from one state to another. On the physical level, sperm and seed connect, germinate, and grow in the warm, dark, watery womb. While on the emotional level, excitement, uncertainty, fear, and dreams mingle interchangeably with one another. In ancient times, midwives were held in great esteem. They were consciously connected to the powerful pulse of the entire cosmos.

In ancient matriarchal times, priests and priestesses trained in healing music would tap deep into the essence of power, through conscious chanting and drumming. Their technology for diving to the inward presence would connect them and their listeners into the wellspring of all that is good. Common archaeological evidence of drums and vocal consciousness practices have been found in the ruins of ancient civilizations that once existed in the modern-day nations of Egypt, Iran, Syria, Israel, and Lebanon.

One example is found in the Hathor Temple complex located in Dendera, Egypt. In this temple, there is a birthing chapel. On the way to the chapel, there are depictions of priestesses on one side of the wall, shown in procession while playing frame drums. On the other side of the wall, they are shown in procession holding sistrums—shakers used in sacred ceremonies—and other ancient percussion instruments.

Birth was assumed to be inherently complicated, requiring professional assistance to increase the chance of neonatal and maternal survival. Pregnant women of all types would come to these chapels, which might be compared to a hospital today, to prepare themselves for the arduous task of birth.

CHAPTER 22

Hearing Miriam's Voice—
and Your Own

Your voice is an instrument. Whether expressed out loud or silently, behaviorally, it is powerful. We tend to pay most attention to the loud voices. But sometimes the soft and quiet ones, or the actions that are observed, are the most penetratingly potent voices.

Miriam's voice made a difference that saved her people from extinction. When Pharaoh decreed the murder of all first-born male children, the Talmud describes how her father, Amram, who was head of the Hebrew community, divorced his wife in response to the decree. Miriam, seeing the folly of this decision, spoke up.

Amram listened to his young daughter and followed her direction. And it happened that his next child was Moses, who would eventually lead their people to freedom from slavery.

It was Miriam who watched over Moses in the bulrushes to assure his safety. It was she who held the vision of transformation for her people. Her voice expressed this power.

Savta Gamila, a widow with five children, fifteen grandchildren, and five great grandchildren, was born to the Druze faith in the Galilee some seventy-five to eighty years ago. (She doesn't know her exact age, as they didn't have birth certificates back in the day). Gamila comes from a long line of herbalist women. Once the medical system was established in the modern state of Israel, she decided to preserve tradition by figuring out a way to incorporate her knowledge of herbs for modern use. She incorporated the special elixirs prescribed by her grandmothers and great-great grandmothers into handmade bars of soap.

As a young woman, Gamila set up a secret laboratory space on the rooftop of her family's home. There, no one would know what she was doing. It was forbidden for a woman to have independent ideas, let alone bring products to market. Today Gamila Secret soaps and skin lotions sell in forty countries around the globe and her factory employs only women: Druze, Jewish, Christian, and Muslim. Her company is a living example of peaceful coexistence. When we met with her our last Feminine Leadership Retreat in Israel, Gamila had recently been awarded a national medal of honor. It is customary for the prime minister to anoint the head of honorees, so he touched hers.

Gamila told our group: "Don't think that once you succeed, you become accepted by your community. Although I've worked for over forty years to honor my religion and tradition, providing work and economic well-being for many, the fact that the prime minister touched my head caused our community to want to run me out of town. In the Druze culture, it is forbidden for a man to touch a woman's head. But I'm not leaving."

As a religious woman, Savta Gamila is voicing her truth and leading the way to bring the value of the Druze religion, steeped in ancient feminine wisdom, into the modern age.

CHAPTER 23

What Is Ancient Wisdom?

The ancients had sophisticated knowledge of science, physics, and the astronomical power of nature, which they harnessed and applied to building the pyramids and other structures that have withstood the sands of time. Recent research studies in the field of archaeo-acoustics are proving this to be true.

Miriam and the other priestesses in ancient Egypt would have been schooled in such knowledge, which they would have used for healing and transformational purposes. The people of the ancient Near East were highly sophisticated in their scientific use of sound and music. They utilized the pentatonic (five-degree) scale and were keen listeners. They used sound in an intuitive way that closely resembled the patterns of the human voice.

Ancient wisdom is based upon the connection of humankind to the cosmos. The ancients understood that there is no separation between the individual and the larger whole. Put another way, the individual is part of the larger mechanism. The individual value of a human being is the importance of the single person's part completing the whole.

Why is this point of view still relevant today? Because we are so disconnected from our inner nature, from one another, and from nature itself. People run around more than ever before trying to accomplish things so that they can feel better about themselves, when what, in fact, they are longing for is connection. Wells used as meeting places have disappeared from the industrialized world. You could argue that the internet is serving to bring people together. I believe that's one of its great gifts. On the other hand, we don't feel as connected when we connect with people through equipment rather than through physical connection.

Returning to the ancient wisdom of simple connection is more important than ever before. This may be one reason why group singing has been on the rise. A recent article in *Time* reported that today, in the United States alone, 32.5 million adults sing in choirs. This is up by almost ten million over the past six years. There are over 270,000 choruses across the country. The article also reports on a recent study that attempts to make the case that "music evolved as a tool of social living."

Our healing music project in the neonatal intensive care unit provided both Israeli and Palestinian mothers to connect to their babies and one another through the therapeutic singing I taught them through our program.

CHAPTER 24

The Kosharot, or Hebrew
Music Goddesses

Earlier, I referred to the Kosharot, ancient Hebrew goddesses who were viewed as the patronesses of wedlock,
birth, and death. Their song (or sung poem) is depicted
in Hebrew writing, on a tablet in the ancient site of Ras
Shamra, located in modern-day Syria. The tablet dates
approximately from the fifteenth or fourteenth century
B.C.E. In January 1938, Theodor Herzl Gaster published
an article in the *Journal of the Royal Asiatic Society:* "The
'Graces' in Semitic Folklore: A Wedding Song from Ras
Shamra."

In this article, Gaster explains that the name K-s-r-t in the poem connects with the Semitic root, Assyrian *keseru*, Hebrew כשר (k-s-r), the primary meaning of which is "to benefit, render blissful, put into proper order," crossed with Arabic (k-t-r), "to be rich, plentiful." From this perspective, the Kosharot may be regarded as the Semitic form of the classical Greek "Charities." It was customary to render thanks to these feminine deities on any occasion of domestic bliss or childbirth.

Part of the function of women standing in for the Kosharot on a special occasion is to stand around and clap hands over the bride, a practice that was designed to frighten away evil spirits thought to hover around the bridal couple. There are Talmudic references to this practice.

There are striking parallels with Old Testament poetry that enhance the importance of this song text. It's also very interesting to note that in the song, the Kosharot are invoked three times. This parallels the well-known Jewish custom of calling three times upon the divine names, such as in the ancient Hebrew prayer: *"Kadosh, kadosh, kadosh"* meaning "Holy, holy, holy."

CHAPTER 25

Feeling and Faith

Now let's look at how the Kosharot song tradition applies to Miriam. There are ten times when we know that the Israelites' experience of redemption found expression through melody and verse. The most well-known of the ten songs of redemption is *Shirat HaYam*, the "Song at the Sea" sung by Moses, Miriam, and the children of Israel upon their crossing of the Red Sea. In the song, they are praising the Divine for delivering them to safety from the pursuing Egyptian army.

There are two versions of the "Song at the Sea," a male and a female version. Why?

The men sang their joy over their deliverance from the Egyptian army being drowned in the sea. They expressed the masculine principle: results and physical outcome. Yet something more was lacking. After the men, the women sang, danced, and played their frame drums to provide it.

What was absent was something beyond the physical results.

What if the men were singing the obvious message and then women were anchoring the powerful essence hiding behind the words? What if their expression were as of the Kosharot? Miriam presided over the female renditions of the "Song at the Sea," with the women collectively expressing the intensity of their fervor and deep faith through their voices in a manner that was unique to the modality of ancient feminine wisdom leadership.

CHAPTER 26

Miriam Led Singing and Dancing

What is not written in the biblical commentary, nor in the Bible itself, is why Miriam led in the singing and dancing of the women in her community. Contemporary understanding of song and dance usually interprets them as displaying the modern sense of celebration. I see something far more significant than just a happy art form. A deeper understanding comes to light if we consider that Miriam may have held a religious office. If she is following the spirit of the Kosharot, the merely celebratory becomes, in that context, an important function.

Add to that the sophisticated knowledge of the scientific use of sound to move matter, and it's not so hard to imagine that Miriam would have been leading with sound and rhythm to alter the physical, psychological, and spiritual states of her people as they were fleeing to freedom. Modern science and quantum physics have proven how sound can move water particles. Look up the video "Amazing Water & Sound Experiment #2" on YouTube and you'll see what I'm referring to.

For me, the parting of seas imagery is an allegory to the notion of birth. *Mitzrayim*, the Hebrew name for Egypt, means "narrow" (as in the birth canal). The parting of the seas is just like parting of the waters in birth. The spiritual realm precedes the physical realm, just as with all manifestation in life. The essence of all matter begins with the primordial waters. The essence of all matter is vibratory. Vibration is sound. Miriam would have understood this.

CHAPTER 27

The Power of Song

The "Song at the Sea" shows us that the courage to change requires having the courage to be different. The Israelites stood at the seashore. It was not until Nachshon—whose name shares the Hebrew root representing the words for *initiation* and *snake* (perhaps referring to kundalini energy?) —took the first step into the sea, that the alchemical magic of molecular shift could occur. He was up to his neck in water already and about to drown when the waters of the Red Sea parted. It was his faith and willingness to go to his death that allowed the miracle to occur.

Miriam, being a prophetess as well as a priestess in the cult of Hathor (as I believe her to have been), would have had her instruments with her at the crossing of the sea. The biblical tale recounts the women singing, dancing, and playing their drums. What would have happened to them in the sea? They would have drowned. No sound could have been made.

What if Miriam, powerful prophetess that she was, trained in the alchemical science of sound, led, using her voice and rhythm to alter the particles of the water? Why not? Medical professionals employ ultrasound to explode kidney stones and aid pregnant women. Opera singers can use their voice to break glass. This too, would have been a conscious use of sound waves.

CHAPTER 28

Standing Up to Authority with Authority

The idea of being driven away from the group can stir up powerful fears. I believe that this explains why we can become so busy inside with weighing our words, thinking about what to say next and how to say it, and worries about how it will sound.

Miriam was punished by God for daring to speak directly to Him. Because of her "transgression," God sent her far away from her camp to live in a leper colony for seven days. What did she experience during that week? She had no one she knew to speak to, no one she trusted with whom to consult, no one she cared for to console her. For someone used to traveling for forty years with the same people, it must have been a terrible ordeal.

How did Miriam support herself through those difficult days when her people shunned her? Was her inner power so firm that she could "turn the other cheek," even when a punishing authority sent her away? Did she accept her fate? Did she rebel? Was she angry? What would her inner dialogue have been? What tools would she have used to calm and nurture herself in such a dire situation, where she was being exposed to a lethal disease? Did she sing and drum or refrain from creatively expressing herself during that time?

Miriam's Source of Power: Self-worth

When she was banished, Miriam must have had feelings come up. It is the human condition. Yet being a spiritual master, she would have been prompted to keep her own counsel and dip deeply into her well of wisdom. This is a story of events that occurred during the period in history when the matriarchal-based feminine worldview was being suppressed. Like anyone whose opinion is suppressed and discounted, to Miriam it must have felt more than uncomfortable to be pushed aside for expressing her honest opinion. On the other hand, Miriam, being connected to her source of wisdom, would have been aware of the monumental changes in the Hebrew culture, so it might not have surprised her much.

One of Miriam's Secrets is that she put herself first—in a feminine way. She was guiding from a deep, cool, calm place. She had no need to shut down her feelings because she was not afraid of the light. She did not need to be seen and heard as a "star," as she knew her worth and was confident of her leadership power. She would not have needed acknowledgment from the "outside" world, because she was rooted deeply to her inner source of power.

What if she used the "timeout" in the leper colony to become even more rooted in her own power? What if she used her isolation to creatively preserve her divine feminine power through the conscious use of music and rhythm?

The Israelites left Egypt with a wealth of knowledge and skills that had been acquired during their sojourn there. If Miriam had been a priestess in the cult of Hathor, the healing art of music would have been one of those skills. It is likely that she was a major keeper of this visceral and intuitive tradition—one based in feminine wisdom and leadership.

But Miriam wasn't really alone. Her people loved and respected her. They valued her presence. We can see evidence of this in the fact that during Miriam's punishment, no one in the Israelite tribe would leave camp without her. Both Moses and his brother Aaron pleaded with God to forgive her. This story, which is recounted in the Numbers 12:15, shows her leadership of her people, including her younger brothers.

CHAPTER 29

Spirit and Matter Are One

I used to believe that spirit and matter did not belong together, a belief common among seekers in some spiritual circles. I was wrong. Quantum science has proven that matter is energy on the subatomic level. Energy is spiritual in its essence. As a spiritual master trained in a feminine religious tradition, the feminine leadership style of Miriam helped to birth a new society for the escaped Hebrew slaves. She was likely a skilled midwife.

Using her special knowledge of how to remain relaxed under pressure and go with the flow, she was able to sustain her feminine power and lead her people through the most tumultuous events of their lives. Her ancient way of approaching life helped ease the pain and discomfort accompanying the process of change they were undergoing, while the new life of the Hebrew culture was being born in the desert. She enchanted the people through her soothing voice and rhythm, which healed the heart and soul of so many who felt at sea, wondering where their journey would take them next.

Contemporary humans have succeeded in overcoming some of the forces of nature. We can split an atom, fly a rocket to the moon, video chat around the planet, and control the temperature in our domiciles. Although we cannot stop an earthquake or a flood, nor can we reverse droughts and feed the starving children living in poverty in Africa, Asia, and elsewhere, we have made tremendous scientific advances during the last 3,000 years. So, you could say that in some ways we have arrived in the Promised Land. Now we need Miriam's guidance and leadership by example to recover the feminine approach to life so that we can transform our competitive approach to one that is nurturing of us all. We need to reclaim our compassion for the tribe that includes all of humanity.

In the next section, we'll explore how we can apply Miriam's lessons in our lives. As we apply what we learn, we can become feminine-style leaders in our personal Promised Lands.

PART 3
CONFIDENCE

Biblical accounts tell of how Miriam had a well that supplied water, sustenance and faith for the Israelites as they wandered through the desert. Her legacy teaches us that when we are going through a process of monumental change, taking time out to replenish ourselves is critical if we are to make it to the finish line. Miriam also teaches us that going slow and steady toward a goal are the actions that give us the stamina to accomplish any goal or intention we set.

Revealing Miriam's Secret

We live in demanding times when it seems as if the entire world is changing. The pace of everything feels like it is speeding up. Structures in our culture that we have relied upon are tumbling at lightning speed. Hierarchical organizations are behind the times. While we are addicted to technology, checking our emails and phones constantly, human engagement has been going haywire. Two people sitting together in a café may well spend more time engaged with their smartphone screens than they do with one another. Yet, despite immense challenges we may be facing personally and collectively, our lives go on day by day.

We must get relief somewhere. If we stop long enough to connect to the inner source, we can discover a deep well of wisdom that can provide answers to any question we may have, including solutions to the most powerful challenges we face.

Change is powerful. It helps us grow and evolve, but it is rarely comfortable or easy. Oppositional thoughts often arise when we try to leave old, destructive habits behind and embrace new, healthier ones. Confusion often stops us when we try to adapt to a new role or situation. Doubt almost always accompanies attempts to learn a new way of being. Others also may oppose us if the changes we are making disrupt their comfortable status quo.

When you're wandering in a territory of not-knowing or conflict within your own mind, you may feel as if you're lost and unsheltered in an arid desert. You may sense you're on the right path, being called forward by a great promise, and yet you may want to lie down and give up. In such times, if you listen closely, a small, compassionate voice that gently murmurs deep inside your heart beckons you to proceed with clarity and courage. This soft, powerful presence guides you to take the next step forward.

Often, the moment we take the next step forward, we meet with inner resistance that feels like a hundred-ton boulder taken from an ancient pyramid. The sound of this conflicting mind warns of imminent danger, directing us to stop dead in our tracks.

Although the supportive, guiding voice speaks so softly that it's almost impossible to hear amid the noise and static of self-will and inner criticism, when we listen to it we can hear this productive mind say, *Where there's a will, there's a way!*

How can we move beyond the resistance? Which voice do we follow?

That's when Miriam's Secret is necessary. The story of Miriam is embedded with lessons on how to create powerful change amid challenge without doing a thing. It is a secret of presence and a way of being that women in the ancient temples of the Near East practiced on a daily basis. Humanity collectively forgot this wisdom long ago as we disconnected from a deeper experience of inner power drawn directly from our ultimate source.

Imagine a physical well for a moment. At the top of the well, the water is clear. At the bottom of the well, the waters are clear. Yet if you dive beneath the surface of the well, you'll stir up silt, mud and debris. This debris muddies the water. At this point, there is no way to separate the mud from the clear water. Yet if you dive deep enough, you get beyond the silt to the clear sweet waters at the bottom of the well.

What if a well of creative power resides silently inside of each of us? This well is the source of our power. What if the Promised Land wasn't a place to find, but instead was the perfect harmony you can only find within yourself? No one can give it to you. You cannot purchase it anywhere. It can only be had by connecting to the source of your power, right inside of you.

When you've got an idea you want to express, that first impulse is pure. It is complete as an idea or dream. Yet if you want to creatively express it or bring it into physical form, you'll meet up with a lot of messiness. Fortunately, if you dive deeply enough and support yourself in being fully present, you end up getting beyond your doubt and confusion. That's the way to gain clarity about what needs to be done. You are then free to act and bring your ideas to fruition.

CHAPTER 30
Still Waters Run Deep

Physical thirst is a metaphor for spiritual longing.

As a deer longs for flowing streams, so my soul
longs for you, O God. My soul thirsts for God, for
the living God.
—Psalm 42

In the text above, thirst carries the deep symbolism of many things: purification, healing, quenching, and the journey from slavery to the Promised Land. Religious texts use the symbol of water to convey a message. In this sense, it can carry divine purpose. Water plays many important roles in religious tasks.

Like the deer that yearns to drink from a stream of clear water, in our hearts we yearn to drink from the well of purity, grace, and femininity.

CHAPTER 31

Birth and Transformation Metaphors Apply to Our Daily Lives

If we look at the story of the Hebrews' flight from slavery to freedom, we can find many parallels in it to personal transformation and to birth. Their thirst for freedom from bondage parallels the deep inner desire for a change of circumstance.

The dream of having a better life often provides us with an inner power to deal with the less-than-dreamy reality of working hard under less than ideal conditions, as the Hebrews fleeing Egypt did, or of living in a way that no longer gratifies us. The dream of the Promised

Land is the sexual, initiating phase of transformation. It's the conception of an idea.

Can we trust what our inner voice of wisdom whispers to us? Can we genuinely live by it? Can we stand up to the authority figures in our lives who would deter us? Will we succeed? These questions signify that we are moving into the pregnancy phase. It's an emotion-filled, watery time.

When Moses met Pharaoh to ask for his people's release, he would have known there was only a one-in-a-million chance Pharaoh would agree. Moses did it anyway. He was gestating the plan that would bring his people to freedom.

In our own lives, we must develop our commitment to the idea of what we are moving toward, just as a woman commits body and spirit to the new life she is bringing into the world. Will I be a good parent to my child? she may wonder. Will we get along? What must I do now so that my baby will be born healthy and thrive?

One of the characteristics of matriarchal energy is that multiple layers of reality coexist. This exemplifies the next phase of birth and transformation.

Although God had parted the waters of the Red Sea, the act of the Hebrews crossing through the waves was like a baby going through the dangerous birth canal. During this transition from the womb to the world, labor contractions cause babies who are being born to experience a flood of emotions, such as fear and excitement, which are mixed together with pain and constriction in an illogical, otherworldly dimension.

It is similar when we are going through personal transformation. Like newborns emerging from the protected realm of water into the unprotected realm of air, all of us must at times cope with the sudden shock of transitioning from one reality to another, with everything that transformation implies. We must leave something behind and let ourselves be transformed if we want to reach the Promised Land of a life we have been envisioning.

Transition is watery and illogical. The path through unknown places may be filled with slippery, dark, and uncertain footing or sudden twists and turns. This can be scary, causing us to recoil to seemingly "solid" ground. We can get stuck simply because it feels safer to stay in the "known" place. Yet, if we don't step outside the comfort zone, we will never get to move to newer ground. But once we're committed to the pregnancy, it's too late to go back. One step in front of the next, one breath after the next, and the actual miracle of birth occurs.

Birth, whether of an actual human baby or of an idea or experience, is our next step. Imagining giving motherly love to our baby and feeling that womb connection helps to prepare us for the intensity of contractions and birthing pains. But we really need a midwife present who is familiar with the passage and can be a safe trusted companion through the process. We need our own Miriam, who as priestess, would have practiced her healing music in the temple, providing solace and wisdom to her people, dreaming with them prior to their departure. We need her skills of prophecy to trust that there is a way to get to our own Promised Land.

In the story of the people who would become the Israelites, Miriam led the women in triumphant refrain for their safe passage through the parted waters, making it possible for new life to begin. The baby was born; arriving safely through the tumultuous birth canal passage. But this is not where their story ends and it is not where our stories end either. The challenges of life demand us to navigate beyond the storms, drawing from our own inner wells of wisdom.

CHAPTER 32

The Relationship Between Literal Birth and Inner Transformation

To explore the relation between literal birth and inner transformation, I met with Mindy Levy, a professional midwife who has assisted in over 1,500 births, both within a hospital environment and in homes. I asked her, "Through all the births you have assisted in, how do you relate birth and transformation?"

Her response was powerful and to the point: "The transformation is the birth of a new self, a changed person, a changed being—someone who has been willing to die in order to be born. It may sound overly simplistic, but every woman I've ever witnessed giving birth or whose birth I have participated in has always undergone some form of transformation. You have to go into hell, then come back to find heaven. If that is not transformation, what is?"

Can you see a correlation to your life? Have you gone through some change where you get to a stage where you think you're going to die? It feels as if you can't go on anymore. When that moment comes, you've just about made it home. As the saying goes "The darkest hour comes just before the dawn."

Levy describes the transformation of women in labor thusly: "There is this movement going on. There are contractions. There's pain. And then there's a rest. It gets more and more painful all the time. Yet the capacity to deal with the pain increases as well. While the pain gets stronger, the hormones released by the body are stronger and they help the woman counteract the pain. As the observing midwife, when a woman says she can't go on, I say to myself, 'Oh good, the baby is on the way.' That's when I know that she is about to give birth.

"When you control your thoughts and emotions, you can actually be going around in circles and not moving ahead." Levy notes. "When the movement becomes chaotic, there is more opportunity for something to break out. From that breaking out, something new can happen. Something new can come in. That is when the transformation occurs." It can be terrifying to surrender to chaos. It feels like all hell is breaking loose.

Drawing upon the well of wisdom inside ourselves is the key to birthing ourselves as we go through life's passages, or when hell is breaking loose and we are trying to manage inner and outer conflict. Finding our inner voice of truth and wisdom is essential to the process of our individual transformation, health, and well-being.

Of course, life is not all smooth sailing once we leave the past behind. There's the period of postpartum, which is full of joy, relief, exhaustion, depression, and another powerful cocktail of emotions. The Israelites postpartum period after escaping bondage in Egypt lasted forty years. That's how long they spent in the desert before they crossed over into their Promised Land.

Although with the advent of the internet, our entire notion of time has sped up, in the grand scheme of things forty years is not all that long a time. The Israelites wandering in the desert were undergoing an entire shift of civilization and worldview. I remember reading somewhere that it required one or two new generations to be born for them to be able to move onwards. New blood. New mentality. It takes time to disengage from one way of being to adopt another.

It is not possible to predict how long any transition in our lives can take us, and yet we must stay the path or fail.

CHAPTER 33

How Can Miriam's Well of Wisdom Help Us in Today's World?

The changes that we experience today are of similar magnitude to those experienced during the times of the Hebrews leaving Egypt, crossing the Red Sea, and wandering through the desert for forty years on their way toward the Promised Land. By taking the time to consider their journey, we can gain wisdom to practice in our own journey to our personal Promised Lands.

What is wisdom really? Wisdom is not something you learn in a book. Wisdom is something gained by years of experience. Each one of us has a unique road to travel in this life. Each person's life brings with it a unique set of lessons. Wisdom is the payoff for all our lessons learned.

> *Keep company with the wise and you will become wise.*
> —*Proverbs 13:20*

When you learn your lessons through life, it is empowering. Your self-worth increases. You treat yourself differently. You end up behaving kindlier toward yourself and others. Others respond to you differently as well.

In ancient times, the elders were highly respected and looked up to. They had lived long enough to learn lessons in life. The wise women were consulted for all kinds of matters.

As you evolve as a human being, as a child of the Divine, your wisdom widens. The more you allow yourself to experience, the more you learn. The more you learn, the more you evolve as a human being. The more you evolve, the wiser you become. The wiser you become, the lighter your experience of life. The lighter your experience of life, the more joy comes in.

Meditating upon the meaning of the word wisdom over the years, I have discovered by intuition an acronym that beautifully sums up its essence. I have come up with different meanings for each of the letters.

Wisdom

W—Worth from Within

I—Intuition = Inside Out

S—Safety and Serenity

D—Dare and Delight

O—Openness and Offering

M—Mothering and Mentoring Yourself

As I continue to meditate upon the letters, my understanding of their meaning shifts and deepens. My wisdom evolves. As you contemplate each of the aspects of wisdom, I invite you to discover your own meaning. No person is the holder of all wisdom for everyone. Answers lie within. Discovering your own wisdom is a beautiful act of self-nurturance. As we take time to listen, we discover new answers and grow our collective well of wisdom.

Let's consider them now in turn.

CHAPTER 34
Worth from Within

When we connect to the source of our collective wisdom, we can discover greater meaning in life. Disharmony, violence, competition, and the illusion of self-sufficiency give way to a shared experience, which supplies meaning. This is the foundation of harmony. This is the way to the Promised Land.

Money comes and goes. Material possessions can be easily lost. Popularity, fame, and being in the "inner circle" in any community or organization can be capricious. True worth is that which cannot be taken away from us by anyone.

While awards, money, big cars, houses, and public acclaim accompany the splashier achievements of some people—even those on a spiritual path—others quietly provide wells of nurturing and support without public attention or commendation. In our modern times, where we have been infatuated with the value of achievement, it's often only when the humble are no longer able to serve that their work is noticed—and then usually only because they are missed for what they helped others to accomplish. The Bible treats Miriam more like the humble worker than the leader I believe she was.

Miriam's ocean of feminine power needed no ranking. She didn't need to win a contest or be the biggest, brightest most popular rock star on the stage. She knew her own worth. She led from the sidelines, regardless of what anyone else had to say about it. She inspired others by her example. This is true leadership.

Her popular status and survivability may have been due to her ability to approach reality from the perspective of the Divine Feminine and the intuitive, emotional, and musical perspective. She attuned herself to the Source of all being. She attuned herself to the Source of the sound of all creation. She was not afraid of the dark and murky waters of the womb space. This allowed her to flow and weave her feminine approach through any and every challenge, even when she was ostracized by God for speaking up.

Unfortunately, many women have not been raised to recognize their intrinsic worth. Even those women

who, like me, came of age during the women's libera-
tion movement of the 1970s find it challenging to
accept ourselves unconditionally. We were raised to
value ourselves according to how much we achieve in
the world. We ourselves viewed the soft and vulnerable
part of us as too weak, something to be overcome instead of embraced.

Men, we are told, experienced a sense of disempow-
erment as more women embraced masculine traits and
perhaps had less need for the opposite sex in their lives.
Fortunately, men and women do not have to be at odds.
The feminine approach lies beyond the male-female
dichotomy: Its embryo lies in the womb of all creation.

CHAPTER 35

Intuition from the Inside Out

Intuition is when you know something from the inside out. Everyone has had an experience of it. Your intuition can speak to you through a variety of ways, often through a gut feeling or strong inner knowing. Think back to those times in your life when you knew something without knowing why or how you knew it. These were examples of your intuition speaking to you. Intuition is a power that comes from deep within your soul; from way beyond your cognitive mind. The intellect cannot make sense of it.

Miriam led intuitively. She needed no how-to book to explain to her how to get things done. There was no precedence for the change that her people were going through. The momentum of societal change then, may be quite like the momentum of change that we are experiencing in the world today. The shift is so drastic that the rules don't apply any more.

Connecting to an inner source of wisdom will provide answers that the intellect cannot provide. As your own prophet, you can ask yourself any question, then go within to listen for the answer. If you will be patient and still, your inner wisdom will guide you.

This is the essence of feminine leadership whose power emanates from the inside out. Try it and discover for yourself.

CHAPTER 36
Safety and Serenity

When you listen to your inner voice earnestly and with clear intention, it creates a sense of safety. Why? Because looking outside of yourself does the opposite: It creates an unconscious sense of insecurity. When you look for safety outside you, your safety depends upon someone or something other than you. It can easily be taken away.

Our entire society is set up around this paradigm of asking: How much money do you make? What kind of car do you drive? What type of computer do you own? What neighborhood do you live in? And on, and on, and on. Thus, we feel insecure a lot of the time.

When you take your answers from within, it creates a different sense, a sense of serenity. No one must tell you what is right or wrong. You know for yourself because you have asked yourself questions such as: "How am I feeling right now?" "What would be the next loving, kind thing for me to do, right this very moment?" Knowing what is right for you to do, be, and have contributes to your inner sense of safety and security. When you feel safe and serene, you are much more open. Your creativity flows.

Besides choosing for yourself what to own, where to live, and how to act, feminine leadership—looking within yourself for answers—means feeling safe to express your truth no matter what others may think or how they might respond.

CHAPTER 37

Dare and Delight

When you dare to follow the wisdom of your heart, it brings untold delight. Daring to act upon your own wisdom, agreeing to follow the direction of your heart, is a powerful and courageous act of leadership. It requires self-trust.

Miriam was a daring leader. She would certainly have been intuitively attuned to the tides of change about to wash over humanity. She dared lead in a way that allowed for experiencing and expressing delight at triumph over difficulty, as evidenced by the Song at the Sea celebration.

And Miriam the prophetess, sister of Aaron, took
a drum in her hand, and all the women went after
her drumming and dancing.
—Numbers 15:20

As you dare to listen to your own wisdom, it will provide answers that you can follow to your Promised Land. As your own prophetess, you understand that you have an inner GPS system that will guide you to a life of delight. That is, if you will truly dare.

CHAPTER 38
Openness and Offering

Once you dare to follow your inner guidance and to delight in the increased self-esteem you'll experience, you will be more open and can offer support to others in trusting their own wisdom. You've got an abundance to give and are open to sharing. Instead of the familiar dynamic of give, give, giving until you're empty and depleted, with nothing left but exhaustion, you've got energy and enthusiasm to share your gifts with the world.

Look at how open Miriam was to offering support. Her well was known for providing both physical and spiritual sustenance to the people in the desert. Nachshon, the first person to walk into the Red Sea, as the

Pharaoh's horsemen pursued the Hebrews from close behind, showed an open offering of faith by literally walking the walk, into the deep waters. His faith opened the way for others to follow suit.

CHAPTER 39

Mothering and Mentoring Yourself

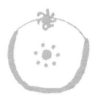

Like a good mother, you can give yourself sustenance whenever you need it. When you are frightened, you need to be nurtured, not pushed into doing more.

Giving results priority over process is a masculine habit. If you are brave, you can brace yourself and push through the fear in any situation. Despite your inner terror, like Superwoman, you move through whatever you must to move forward. The problem is that this habit requires you to expend lots of energy, so you can become worn out. If you are fearful, you may bolt. Or instead of speaking up, you silence yourself and defer your judgment to others'. Perhaps you don't make an important phone call or don't respond to a jabbing re-mark that humiliates you for fear of making things worse. It's the fight-or-flight syndrome at work.

An alternative way to meet your terror or respond to stress in your life is to mother yourself. This means allowing space and time for things to be and evolve as they naturally do. When you mother yourself, you be-come the mentor to your own capabilities. Your mentorship allows space for your vulnerable side to heal and transform with the attention of the most im-portant person in your life . . . YOU!

Antoine de Saint Exupéry writes: "What makes the desert beautiful is that somewhere it hides a well." What makes you beautiful is that the nurturing mother principle is right inside of you, waiting for you to drink from it.

CHAPTER 40

Connect to the Soft, Silent Power Within

If the soft, fluid, intuitive approach sounds appealing to you, you can learn to make peace with yourself through connecting with silence. By listening to yourself, you will be able to hear what is truly important to you; this brings with it a sense of safety and security. Taking time to listen to yourself puts you into contact with your true power. It returns you to the Now moment from which you are always able to consciously choose what is best for you. From this "place," you are better able to focus, which then helps you to function joyfully in any field of endeavor.

The intense power of Miriam's silent voice and constant attention to the rhythm of life provided a safe container—a well—to connect to the same benevolent divine power that led her people safely to freedom. The moment of passage from slavery, through the treacherous, parted seas and out into the wilderness, was marked by Miriam's musical praise, a song of celebration. Similarly, you can celebrate the moments of your divine connection and safety every day.

As the Hebrews wandered through the wilderness, lacking adequate water would have been fatal. The power of Miriam's integrity, caring, and loving kindness was such that the Divine provided a moving well of water, one which followed the people throughout their wanderings until the moment of her death. Without Miriam, who represented the Mother Principle for her people, there would have been no water.

While male prophets emphasize the power of words, the centrality of rules of conduct, of sanctity, and of justice, Miriam's prophecy was a display of silent power. Rather than stirring speeches or administration of justice, she taught her people how to consciously use their voices and rhythm to connect with the Divine. This helped them to prosper during a period of exposure and fragility, wandering hundreds of miles in the wilderness for decades trying to find the right place to make their home.

It is important for us to remember that in biblical times in the ancient Near East, the worldview was feminine in nature, characterized by a nonlinear, nonrational character.

A problem we in the Western world face is that when we try to generate change or to create something new, whether by using manifestation principals, positive thinking, meditation, or any other technique, we tend to approach reality as a "doer." From this perspective, we would never be able to get to the essence of the matter, even if we meditated twenty-four hours a day.

The essence of successful change or creation lies with the Source. Source is beyond mind. That means that to find deeper meaning, you've got to be willing to go "out of your mind." That is a scary notion for the intellect, which loves to stay in charge.

Transformation from a feminine perspective requires no doing. There's nothing to be done. Instead, it requires us to connect to the soft, fluid, intuitive approach of being. It requires us to be our own companions, our own prophetesses, if you will.

CHAPTER 41

Listen to Yourself

The worst form of cruelty is not hatred, but indifference. With hatred, you know where you stand. Indifference is a total lack of acknowledgement of worth.

When we do not listen to our inner voices, we ignore ourselves. How do children react when you ignore their needs? They whine, they act up, they act out, or they do whatever else they need to do to get your attention. When you do not listen to yourself in earnest, underneath the surface, those parts will act out in other ways to get your attention. If you are pushing yourself too hard, doing too much, not stopping, your body will become sick to get your attention.

Taking the time to listen to yourself is a loving act, even when it is just for a few moments. When you pay attention, you can take care of your true inner needs. The basic physical need for sufficient rest is often dishonored today. And lack of sleep will disrupt your entire system. Listening connects you to the actions related to your wellness, such as slowing down and resting. Slowing down can be the fastest route to any destination.

No matter what the circumstances of your life are, no matter where you are in the process of birthing a transformation, it is important to remember that you are an instrument of creation. Attuning to the silence of the well within you will connect you with the soft side of life, the generator of all that is good in your Promised Land.

CHAPTER 42

Creating Without Doing a Thing

Let's go back to the "official" story of the Hebrew exile, to see how the Divine Feminine principle expresses itself through the story of Miriam. Remember the scene of the young woman standing watch in the bulrushes at the edge of the Nile, rooted in her faith, persevering even in the face of Pharaoh's persecution? (Exodus 2:4) She watches over her brother from afar while tapping into an inner source of power. She waits quietly. Living fully absorbed in the present moment, she has no need to plan. She knows.

Miriam is guided by divine inspiration. She trusts and listens for signs. Meeting the Pharaoh's daughter and suggesting that Moses' own mother serve as his wet nurse is a perfect example of her ability to create without "doing" a thing. Her success occurs naturally and flows without incident.

Wouldn't you love to be able to do that?

In the modern world, our focus upon achievement teaches us to be the doer. The classic image propagated by the novels of Horatio Alger a century ago teaches us that it is the power of the individual's actions that determine his value, not how he came into this world. Alger wrote over one hundred boys' stories about impoverished children with nothing but a few pennies in their hands who bettered their circumstances through hard work and perseverance.

In American culture, the person who is born with nothing and achieves against all odds is valued even more than the one born into riches. I'm not suggesting for a moment that there is anything wrong with building a business empire, earning a fortune, or even working diligently. The problem is that we have been taught to equate freedom and the pursuit of happiness with "doing."

We have become disconnected from the simple pleasure of our being through:

- Competing goals.
- Competing commitments.
- Overworking.
- Stressing.
- Not having enough time for ourselves.

Accepting the freedom not to do? That's considered confrontational.

The modern worldview values activity over stillness. We even try to "achieve" spiritual enlightenment. To regain some balance in our lives, it is important for us to reconnect to ourselves. This requires slowing down and relaxing more often. In ancient times, this was practiced as a matter of course. Time was taken every day to reflect.

The voices in our head are not seen, and yet we experience them as being very powerful. When we quiet our minds, we are dipping into the well.

CHAPTER 43

The Tongue Is Mightier Than the Sword

Negative words often arise in awareness from the subconscious reaches of our minds.

How do you think Miriam would have dealt with negative self-talk? I suppose she would have dealt with it by turning inward. She was schooled in the alchemical power of sound, whose source is silence, so she would have known how to transform the silt of her critical internal voices into the soothing balm of healing song, for instance.

The need to belong is so intense at times that sometimes we even go against ourselves just to fit in. Fear, anger, anxiety, and confusion can stop us from expressing what we truly feel. We tend to practice "politically correct" behavior even if it goes against our grain. We smile and speak pleasantly, even if we're seething with anger and would rather blow off steam. While we remain pleasant, our behavior toward ourselves then can turn violently self-negating.

If you criticize yourself, you run the risk of damaging your self-esteem. It doesn't matter how successful you are. All the millionaires and movie stars who have committed suicide at the peak of their careers attest to the potency of negative self-talk. Although such people have achieved what most people dream of, perhaps believing that when they got them, then they would be "worthy enough," "likeable enough," or "lovable enough" to others, no outward show of success could ever have been as important as valuing themselves.

CHAPTER 44

Overcoming Negative Self-talk

What if your success was a function of how you speak to and support yourself inside the private well of your inner psyche? How often do you feel listened to and truly heard? How important is this to you? Are you "drinking" clear, cool, refreshing "water" or poisoning yourself with the subtle, yet destructive "liquid arsenic" of self-censorship?

I have discovered that people's ability to express their unique gifts in the world and enjoy the fruits of their labor is closely linked to how well they meet and respond to their own negative self-talk.

We are the ones whose approval we are looking for. So why don't we just stop and listen to ourselves? What could be simpler? Perhaps the gift of ignoring our authentic voices is that when we've finally had enough pain and suffering, we surrender. When we surrender, we are free to listen. We can follow the whispers of our hearts and souls, which provides u with a deep sense of fulfillment and satisfaction. Perhaps this explains why surrender is called sweet.

The healing essence of sound is rooted in the silent gap that lies just beyond the conscious mind. When we go to connect to the source of harmony, sometimes we encounter the exact opposite of it. It is not comfortable to meet up with disharmony.

Most of us do not revel in discovering our dark side that lurks deep within. At the slightest wink of discomfort, we run like the devil. We judge, criticize, and deflect our inner discomfort outwardly. We stay in our heads and disconnect from our feelings. We explain our feelings away. In doing so, we never get to enjoy a true sense of satisfaction and fulfillment.

CHAPTER 45

Self-compassion Increases Power

We have become so out of contact with our nature, living from an intellectual worldview, that it takes reconnecting to forgotten parts of ourselves that lie beyond our conscious understanding to reconnect to our full nature. These parts, which are resistant, unwilling, petulant, and defensive, reside in the layer of silt beneath our intellectual shields. Silt, when mixed with the flow of water, is penetrable. This means that our defensive shields soften through self-compassion, allowing for constructive life energy to be released and transformed into powerful expression. They hold gifts if they are met with gentleness and kindness.

Inner transformation happens when we are courageous enough to dig into our well of unconscious silt. If we are willing to acknowledge the less than savory parts of our personalities, we are empowered to come to a deeper place of self-acceptance. With self-acceptance also comes an increased sense of self-compassion.

Receiving self-compassion is a powerfully acknowledging experience.

Authentic power needs no acknowledgement from the outside. An inner sense of knowing provides all the authenticity you need. Then if you also receive validation from the outside, it is like a cherry on top of the whipped cream on top of the ice cream sundae.

CHAPTER 46

Reconnecting to Your Source

How do you get to the well inside? How can you reconnect to your authenticity?

Be willing to dive into the moss-filled crevices of your inner life—even if you might be more comfortable leaving them sunken and unexposed.

The bottom-line process is so simple: Stop. Do nothing. Honestly listen to yourself.

Honestly.

Compassionately.

Are you enslaving yourself through overthinking everything you do and repeatedly questioning yourself, or by looking to others for your answers instead of listening deeply for your own inner truth? Then try an exercise to quiet yourself and create harmony.

I discovered this technique when I was particularly overwhelmed one day with overlapping commitments and too little time to complete them. I went into my own well of wisdom and the results were surprising. A profound healing ensued.

First, go with the flow. Wanting to change reality is a sure way to create dissonance. The place where you feel the biggest block is the most powerful place to stop pushing.

Second, meet your critical voices with compassion. Whether you find your negative chatter chiding you for transgressing some invisible unwritten rule, or behaving in a manner you find embarrassing, see if you can just listen, without reacting defensively or trying to change it. Compassion goes a long way to melting the frigid ice of inner attack. You will be delighted to discover your outer world becoming more harmonious as well.

CHAPTER 47

Encountering Resistance

When going through a process of change or transformation, your old mode of thought or behavior must die or be abandoned to give way to a new way of being. Change does not occur in an orderly fashion. Life has its own agenda and own way of operating. Even with your best efforts at positive thinking or using the law of attraction, many times what you intend and the results you hope for just don't come to fruition. Why? Is there something wrong with you? Is your negative behavior getting in the way? The randomness of some outcomes may cause you to doubt your ability to change. Yet many times, a hidden mode of existence is in operation.

Underneath our conscious mode of operating, lies a deeper source of power. This area is dominated by the feminine principal, receptivity. These are the untidy, murky waters of the womb, which has the capacity to create life. Creative receptivity is invisible to the eye, unperceivable by our masculine-dominated intellects, which cannot understand its mechanisms. Dwelling in the underworld of gestation can be accompanied by confusion due to a lack of clear-cut boundaries and logical perceptions. To the linear functions of the conscious mind, the territory of the subconscious mind might feel ominous and dangerous. What we cannot understand triggers a fear of the unknown.

If we feel nervous, instead of prophetically seeing our success up ahead and acting as patient midwives to ourselves as we slowly go through the process of change, we may bolt and run before our worthy ideas and intentions can crystallize into form in physical reality. We never reach the Promised Land of which we dreamed.

Seeing pain as a natural part of the process of personal transformation enlarges our perspective. Otherwise we might think of pain only as a sign of pathology or a stigma. This new outlook permits us to have empathy for our suffering and view it as a natural aspect of healing. It permits suffering to gestate a new solution in its own way and its own time.

Healing occurs when we're being receptive, because the process of life is given attention by an empathetic presence. Any mirroring situation in our lives that touches this pain, wherever it shows up, shows us that we are all right, even in our imperfection. The process unfolds of its own accord and ends our silent suffering. We learn that it is OK not to be perfect.

CHAPTER 48

Melting Resistance

When you assert your integrity, even when it seems that old habits, your history, or others are against you, the universe hears your call. Outside, in the physical world, it may look as if everything is falling apart. The way you have operated up until now may no longer work. Doing more, working harder, making more effort is all connected to that masculine "doing" side of existence. When change is occurring, focusing energy outward is not so effective. Shifting your focus inward is. At those times when you are at your wit's end, you are still with yourself. It is then when calling to the well within you can be of special importance.

One of the most powerful things you can do to discover your inner well of wisdom during times when the world pushes back at you, is to slow down and connect. At these times, it's not what you do that is so important, but rather what you don't do. There is a well-known saying, attributed to Benjamin Franklin, "When the well's dry, we know the worth of water." This perhaps is another way of offering us an opportunity to value simple things more, like the simple pleasures of life and friendship and kindness—particularly self-kindness. To do so, we might learn much from revaluating our lives in accordance with our principles. The contrast between opposites can teach us.

When you listen to the voice of wisdom inside you during periods of pressure or rapid change, instead of responding through habit, you tap into the source of your true power. You fill your well with the water and discover the ability to divine any answer to any question you could possibly ask. It just requires the willingness to stop and listen internally for the answer.

The closer you get to the source of your true power, the more your own resistance to change may flare up. When you dare to express your deepest desires, a fear of making waves, creating disturbance, or receiving disapproval (your own or that of another), can keep you from following through on what you know to be best for you. When you do not follow through, you violate yourself. Because you disconnect from your power, you stop good from flowing to you.

Allowing space and time for things to "be" is the feminine principle at work. It is like allowing time for a seed to spout. If you dig in the dirt every day to look at the seed, a plant will never grow to fruition. Yet, allowing things to be in our world of immediate results is all too often considered lazy, irresponsible, or unimportant. The internet has created a dynamic where our attention is so divided that it exacerbates the need to be "bigger, better, and more dazzling" just to be seen and heard for a moment. Leaving things alone to germinate on their own may seem akin to social suicide. Some see this approach as weak and ineffective.

If you avoid letting things be, you will never get to experience the deep sense of satisfaction that comes from experiencing the nonlinear and uncontrollable process of creation. Choosing to trust and consciously allowing for the process to unfold enables powerful results to come to full fruition. Supposedly, Mahatma Gandhi said, "Be the change you wish to see." The point is well taken. Being as you intend to be—if it is not what you are yet—requires you to have the willingness to create waves, learn to think differently, and challenge your comfortable habits.

It is said that Miriam's well provided nourishment in the desert. In those times when there was nothing to eat, its water provided the people with sufficient nourishment to get them through their difficulties. It was their faith in the beneficence of a higher source that pulled them through. Symbolically, Miriam's well represents a soft power that can ease the prickly, pointing jabs of difficulty and the controlling energy we meet inside us when we want to change the reality of whatever is going on in our lives. This well can help us consciously connect with a different type of nurturance. It provides confidence, resolve, and inner balance.

CHAPTER 49

Flow into Your Promised Land

Miriam believed in the transformation her people were experiencing on the way from living in slavery to freedom in the Promised Land, even when others didn't. She was patient. She knew how to live in the gray areas of life, outside the clearly defined habits of black and white rules. What can we learn from her? What can we gain?

From Miriam, we can learn to be truly centered in self. Self-centeredness has gotten a bad rap, particularly as it pertains to women. If a woman takes care of her needs first, she may be called a bitch. She may be thought of as selfish or insensitive to the needs of others.

This couldn't be further from the truth.

You cannot be giving if you ignore giving to yourself. If you are insensitive to your needs, how could you possibly be responsive to someone else's needs? You greedily hold back the abundant gifts that you were born to share. Then you lack the means to support whatever it takes to show up at your best. Asking for more may bring up the fear of rejection or criticism. The intent of the Divine is for us to share our voices, not to hold them back. Sharing our authentic voices is one of the main reasons for being alive. It is "good" selfishness when you ask for what you truly need so you can share your unique talents in the highest way possible. Your example teaches strength, courage, openness, and abundant prosperity to others. When you have more than enough to give and you share it, good grows. Everyone wins. There is enough to go around. Your example inspires others to show up for themselves, like you are doing.

I recently worked with a client to help her stop holding back from expressing her truth. Following her father's death, she committed to step up and "own" her leadership role. At sixty-two years old, it was time to lead with her feminine power.

During a private immersion retreat with me, this woman found her authentic voice and established a power map for her personal and professional goals. After connecting to her ancient roots on our annual feminine leadership journey in Israel she courageously announced her plans to her family: She would now act on her lifelong dream to found a home birthing center.

Upon returning home to the United States, my client took the risk to voice her vision to the city council of her town and they expressed interest in collaborating with her to establish a countywide service. She's now on her way to building a sustainable income for herself, and for the many people the center will employ to deliver birthing services.

All this occurred because she dared to stop holding back, decided to say yes, and acted upon the instructions of her inner authority.

Like my client, Miriam acted upon her own authority. From a masculine world perspective, this might be viewed as "being uppity." Who are you to speak up for yourself and trust in your inner direction? In the biblical account, God punished Miriam harshly, sending her away from the tribe to isolation in the leper colony. Many men and women fear something similar.

Is being rejected or ousted from a group a fear that keeps you from speaking up for yourself? Miriam was trained as prophetess within a society that had been rooted in a feminine worldview for thousands and thousands of years. Therefore, she understood her power. According to biblical writers, she acted against the consensus view. But I think they got it wrong. Despite the punishment, Miriam accepted herself—and this had impact. The people would not leave camp without her. Moses and Aaron pleaded for God to spare her. She had an authentic power that caused even the leader of the nation to depend upon her leadership.

Masculine energy upholds the law and the ways we behave in society. Feminine energy and wisdom within provide us a source of power. It is the very essence of life that emanates from within that is this source. Without inner wisdom, outer laws are empty shells with empty action.

Today, more than ever, it is helpful to reconnect to our inner well of wisdom as it can provide the bridge from our inner truth to our outer actions. This is the essence of right living and it creates harmony.

I believe that Miriam's clear connection to her inner well of wisdom is why the Israelites would not leave without her. They recognized that she provided them access to the unseen source of their security. That unseen, oceanic power lying deep within enabled the ragged group of former slaves to stay committed while they crossed a dry stretch of desert to arrive at the Promised Land.

What worked before in the "old country" would no longer be effective or efficient in the new reality they were moving toward. Not being willing to let go of the old ways, even if comfortable, would have kept them slaves forever. Their vision had to motivate them.

Do you believe it is selfish to express yourself directly or to seek satisfaction? Perhaps it seems hedonistic.

Do you believe, "A caring and kind person puts others first"? Perhaps you reason with yourself: "After all, these times are hard, and indulgent thinking is inappropriate."

Maybe you wonder, "Who am I, to put my authentic desires first?"

When you don't listen to the authentic calling of your inner voice of wisdom, you are shutting off your power and shutting out your good. Fortunately, there is no limit to good, and the universe will always give you another chance. Yet sometimes, the gifts you have to give and those you receive are meant for one point in time only. If you do not allow yourself to receive them, or to give them, you won't get to reap their rewards.

Do you deprive yourself of your personal Promised Land by keeping yourself a slave of "efficiency," doing, doing, doing until you drop from exhaustion?

Miriam's well provided sustenance for an entire people. Her authentic voice and rhythm allowed everyone in her community to be seen and heard. The fact that her people refused to move along without her proves the power of the modalities she would have employed to lead them. When people gather together and each voice is expressed and heard, this forms a unified whole, a living garden of Eden. Everyone is nourished. This is an expression of true abundance and prosperity.

When we connect to our inner truth and express it, positive change occurs.

ACKNOWLEDGMENTS

My first and foremost thanks is to the Higher Power that brought me here with my parents as vehicles.

Thanks to the prophetess Miriam, and goddesses Sekhmet and Hathor, whose feminine leadership nurtures and teaches me inner acceptance and power.

So many people have contributed to my life and made this book possible. Friends, clients, and students have all contributed to my practicing the concepts and using the tools presented in this book. Heartfelt thanks to you all.

Special mention goes to Lester Levenson, who taught me to look inside of myself for answers, Annrika James who taught me the Sedona Method, Paramahansa Yogananda, who has chaperoned me across the continents, and Amarananda Bhairavan (Nandu), who confirmed my inner knowledge regarding ancient Hebrew feminine power, and through whose spiritual mentorship I made the commitment to share this material when the appropriate time came.

Also, I am grateful to:

- Stephanie Gunning, who helped me craft the original concept of this book and showed me how to hone my message, and also guided the physical production of the book.

- Jacqueline Simmonds, who recognized that *Miriam's Secret* was a series of four books.
- Vanessa Squire Kaliski, Maryanne Savino, Tzipi Radonsky and Janis Gildin for their helpful editorial eyes.
- Marianne Williamson, Byron Katie, and Doron Kit Foster and Victoria Davies for cover design.
- Bella Shahar Hillel for the front cover photograph.
- Libshtein, a powerful Israeli mentor embodying the divine feminine power of Israel.
- Molly Gordon and Mark Silver who introduced me to the ethical, authentic means of marketing online, founded in spiritual truth.
- Jonathan Fields, Jayme Johnson, Wendy Keller, and Christine Kloser, who taught me the skills of book crafting and marketing them.
- My cousin Sharon Weil who asked me who I want around my well.
- The healing musicians, sound healers and many frame drum groups and teachers who are helping to revive an important ancient art.
- Marilyn Stern, Michal Noam, Angela Deger, David Milton and Dwight Fortune for their support and friendship.

BIBLIOGRAPHY

Joan Cook. "Wells, Women, and Faith," *Proceedings of the Eastern Great Lakes and Midwest Biblical Societies,* volume 17 (1997), pp. 11–18.

William G. Dever. *Did God Have a Wife? Archaeology and Folk Religion in Ancient Israel* (Grand Rapids, MI.: Eerdmans, 2008).

Ellen Frankel and Betsy Platkin Teutsch. *The Encyclopedia of Jewish Symbols,* (Woodstock, VT.: Skylight Paths Publishing, 2005).

Theodor Herzl Gaster, "The 'Graces' in Semitic Folklore: A Wedding Song from Ras Shamra," *Journal of the Royal Asiatic Society* (January 1938).

The Jewish Encyclopedia. Available at: http://jewishencyclopedia.com.

New World Encyclopedia. Available at: http://newworldencyclopedia.org.

Raphael Patai. *The Hebrew Goddess, third enlarged edition* (Detroit, MI.: Wayne State University Press, 1990).

W. Gunther Plaut and David E.S. Stein. *The Torah: A Modern Commentary, revised edition* (New York, N.Y.: Union for Reform Judaism Press, 2005).

Alison Roberts. *Hathor Rising: The Power of the Goddess in Ancient Egypt* (Rochester, VT.: 1997).

Rami Shapiro, translator. *The Divine Feminine in Biblical Wisdom Literature* (Lanham, MD.: Rowman and Littlefield Publishers, Inc, 1992).

VOICES OF EDEN RESOURCES

Stay connected with Eliana Gilad and the Voices of Eden Project via the website www.voices ofeden.com.

Also connect with Eliana through the Institute's Facebook page: www.facebook.com/healing voice.

If you would like Eliana to speak to your group, she is available in person or via Skype or conference call. Please contact her at speaker@voicesofeden.com to arrange an appearance.

We invite you to join us for the Voicing Your Feminine Power and Wisdom Live Online Training, a program designed for successful women suffering with self-doubt. The training helps women build the confidence they need to fully share their passion and power with the world. Find all the details at www.voicesofedenlive.com.

If you're ready for a life-changing travel experience, consider the Ancient Wisdom Feminine Leadership Retreat to Israel. For a description and more details, visit www.voicesofedenlive.com.

ABOUT THE AUTHOR

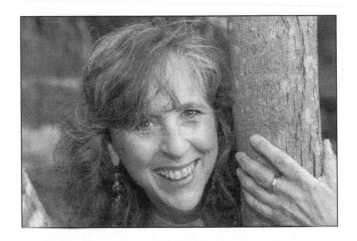

Eliana Gilad is a TEDx presenter, motivational speaker, teacher, composer, and performer, and founder of Voices of Eden Ancient Wisdom and Healing Music Institute. Born in the United States, Eliana left for France in 1991 and then moved to Israel in 1994. Professionally, she has dedicated her life to reviving the conscious use of voice and rhythm as natural healing instruments, as they were used in ancient matriarchal times. This wordless healing sound modality helps people find their authentic voices and connect to their inner calm and wisdom. It has been clinically researched in a neo-natal intensive care unit, where it was proven to lower blood pressure and heart rate, increase focus, and improve the quality of sleep. Her work has been featured in publications like *Drummer, Yoga Journal, Mothering, Music and Medicine Journal, Global Rhythm,* and *Hindustan Times.* Documentarian Emmanuel Itier also features Eliana in her award-winning film *Femme* (2013), narrated by Sharon Stone.

Eliana is a frequent keynote presenter, teacher, and performer at healing music, leadership, health, and mindfulness conferences throughout the world. Such events include TEDxSanJuan (2017), International Conference of Traditional Music (2017), Globe Sound Healing Conference (2014), TEDxVailWomen Conference (2012), Chinese Spa Conference (2011), Music and Medicine Symposium (2010), and Legends of Non-violence Conference (2007). She has also presented at the United Nations, the Chopra Center in New York City, and the Thank Water Conference (2003), alongside Masaru Emoto, author of *Messages from Water,* whose research revealed the profound effect of her music upon frozen water molecules.

Through her Institute, Eliana researches and teaches the principles of feminine power and the voice. She is the author two previous books: *Rhythms of the Natural Voice Workbook* and *Quiet in the Eye of the Storm: Living Peace in a War Zone,* written during the 2006 Israeli-Lebanon War. She has produced five music CDs and a groundbreaking relaxation music program used by dentists worldwide. Eliana also narrated the "The Forgotten Jews," a PBS documentary broadcast in November 2005. In 1992, she broadcast the voiceovers for CBS television during the Winter Olympics in Albertville, France.

She alternately makes her home in Los Angeles, California, and Galilee, Israel.

Made in the USA
San Bernardino, CA
06 September 2017